Imaging Science

Imaging Science

Peter Carter, M.A., B. Ed. (Hons), Cert. Ed., F.C.R., T.D.C.R.
Formerly Principal Lecturer
Sheffield Hallam University

Blackwell
Science

© 2006 by Blackwell Science

Blackwell Publishing Ltd
Editorial offices:
Blackwell Science Ltd, 9600 Garsington Road, Oxford OX4 2DQ, UK
   Tel: +44 (0) 1865 776868
Blackwell Publishing Inc., 350 Main Street, Malden, MA 02148-5020, USA
   Tel: +1 781 388 8250
Blackwell Science Asia Pty Ltd, 550 Swanston Street, Carlton, Victoria 3053,
Australia
   Tel: +61 (0)3 8359 1011

First published 2006

ISBN-13: 978-06320-5656-9
ISBN-10: 0-6320-5656-8

Library of Congress Cataloging-in-Publication Data
Carter, P. H. (Peter H.)
   Imaging science / Peter Carter.
      p. ; cm.
   Includes bibliographical references and index.
   ISBN-13: 978-0-632-05656-9 (pbk. : alk. paper)
   ISBN-10: 0-632-05656-8 (pbk. : alk. paper)
1. Diagnostic imaging.
   [DNLM: 1. Diagnostic Imaging–methods. 2. Diagnostic Imaging–
instrumentation.   WN 180 C324i 2006] I. Title.

   RC78.7.D53C38   2006
   616.07′54–dc22

A catalogue record for this title is available from the British Library

Set in 10 on 12.5 pt Palatino
by SNP Best-set Typesetter Ltd., Hong Kong
Printed and bound in Singapore
by Fabulous Printers Pte Ltd

For further information on Blackwell Publishing, visit our website:
www.blackwellpublishing.com

Contents

Acknowledgements

I am indebted to all the students I met and tried to help as a lecturer, but particularly to those who openly admitted, 'I don't understand this . . .' or complained, '*Why* are we having to learn this . . .?'. I offer them this textbook, in a belated attempt to prove that their efforts were worthwhile.

I have depended heavily on expert input from clinical specialists in the fields of computed tomography (Ann Heseltine), magnetic resonance imaging (Gail Darwent), ultrasound imaging (Ann Allen and Elaine McInnes), computed radiography (Julian Dean) and radionuclide imaging (Andrew Hyatt). I must record my special thanks to them, and add a note of extra appreciation to Andrew for his assistance with the book as a whole. Other clinical specialists who have been kind enough to offer constructive criticism of the text have included Edna White, Rowan Spriggs and Gerard Nowak.

I am especially grateful to my wife, Sheila, for her patience in accepting that a book cannot be written without disruption of domestic calm and order.

Finally – and, if the others will allow me, most of all – I must record my sincere gratitude to the publishers and all their colleagues at Blackwell Publishing. They have demonstrated an extreme and infinite degree of patience, when faced with wave after wave of disappointment and delay. This is their book as much as mine.

Peter Carter, Sheffield

Introduction

In 1895, Roentgen's historic discovery of X-rays launched diagnostic medical imaging – a service that has saved the lives of millions of patients and, reinforced by a century of progress, continues to do so today. The significance of this new discovery was immediately recognised; it was used widely and enthusiastically. But as time passed, some latent hazards become apparent: it was discovered that X-ray exposures could trigger changes within the body's cells, altering their function and possibly proving fatal.

Medical imaging science addresses these conflicting issues, and this book aims to encourage students to adopt as central features of their own practice:

- improving image quality, to ensure maximum diagnostic information,
- minimising potential harm to patients during their imaging examinations, and
- eliminating all danger to staff.

Chapters 1-5 cover X-ray imaging, from conventional procedures through to computed tomography (CT). Especially for readers whose previous studies of physical science have been limited, commentary notes, recognisable by their grey background, accompany the main text of the first four chapters. These offer definitions of terms, explanation of principles and discussion.

Three further chapters explain the imaging modalities based on gamma radiation (RNI), ultrasound and nuclear magnetic resonance (MRI). Technically, specialised imaging modalities stand well apart from conventional X-ray imaging. This fact has tended to exclude them from the early years of a radiography curriculum. But now, as their availability expands, first-choice use of CT, RNI, MRI and ultrasound imaging suggests that students should learn about them sooner. Chapters 5–8 have been specially written as introductions to these modalities' principles and vocabularies.

Throughout the book, the burden of facts and figures has been deliberately limited; the aim has been to adopt a 'light touch'. Opinions may differ on what needs to be known (or not), about some topics. For example, though automated equipment's time and labour-saving facilities unquestionably benefit patients and staff alike, they raise an important question for students and those concerned with their education. If equipment is modelled on the 'Just switch on and use!' principle, to what extent should the saved time and labour be devoted to learning the secrets behind its automation? Anxious reactionaries will insist on deep and thorough study. Liberated technophobes will simply keep the service engineer's telephone number handy. This book tries to follow a pragmatic course. I hope readers will find it accessible rather than daunting, and interesting rather than boring. It can, of course, be treated as a quick-access resource for coping with the temporary challenges posed by exams and assignments. But longer-term use is suggested as preferable – particularly if what it offers is integrated with other learning resources: complementary textbooks, journals, research papers, official reports and the increasingly huge range of facilities available via the Internet.

Above all, if it helps to bring benefits to some of your patients and reduce the risks to others, its writing – and your reading – will have been worth the effort.

Chapter 1

A survey of X-ray imaging

The nature and properties of X-radiation

X-rays form part of a spectrum of radiant energies, known as the **electromagnetic radiations**, (Figure 1.1) grouped together because of their common properties. These include travelling at the same, constant velocity and the ability to cross a vacuum. But each also has its own special properties: *infra-red radiation* alone is perceived as 'hot', for example, and only *light* is visible.

Here are some properties of X-radiation.

Selective penetration

The ability to pass through structures and substances isn't limited to X-rays: microwaves carrying mobile phone messages, and radio waves can penetrate buildings. But when X-rays travel through a structure, they can be uniquely affected by even the slightest variations in its composition. This property is essential for creating an X-ray image's **contrast**.

Straight-line propagation (travel)

All electromagnetic radiations have this property. It is significant to the diagnostic use of X-rays in giving reliability to radiographic images: objects placed in the path of an X-ray beam cast shadows that retain their shape. When absorbent barriers are used to provide

Electromagnetic radiations

Electromagnetic radiations are so called because they are formed by transverse vibrations of electric and magnetic fields. They can be thought of as continuous energy waves, but it is probably easier to understand X-ray production and interactions if an alternative model is used, regarding an X-ray beam as a flow of energy packets, *photons*.

Contrast

By penetrating objects to a greater or lesser extent, an X-ray beam produces the familiar black-and-white patterns recognised as X-ray images. But an image is very rarely composed, literally, of black and white alone; there are also numerous shades of grey. The term *contrast* is used to indicate how distinctly an image identifies adjacent structures, translating them into different steps along a scale of grey tones or densities. A high-contrast image contains a wide range of tones (from black through to white); a low-contrast image is confined to a restricted range of grey tones.

Speed of light

This is the term used to describe the common velocity of all electromagnetic radiations. It could equally well be termed 'the speed of X-rays' – or of radio waves, etc. but visible light gets the vote because of its familiarity. It is inconceivably fast: three hundred million metres per second ($3 \times 10^8 \, \text{m s}^{-1}$) so, for all practical purposes, X-ray exposures start and stop instantly: there is no build-up or fade-away.

Energy

Energy exists everywhere, in many familiar forms: food, heat, sound, light, etc. The *Law of Conservation of Energy* states the thought-provoking fact that, within a defined system, *energy cannot be created and cannot be destroyed*; but it allows that energy can be converted from one form to another. This is well illustrated by the

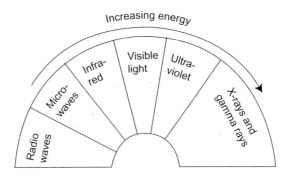

Figure 1.1 Spectrum of electromagnetic radiations.

radiation protection, the radiation's predictable, straight path enables them to be positioned accurately and effectively.

High velocity

The high velocity of all electromagnetic radiations (the '**speed of light**') makes the production of X-ray images instantaneous: they immediately record the patient's observed position, phase of respiration, etc., without the complication of a delay.

Ionisation

When materials are exposed to an X-ray beam, they absorb some of its **energy**. During the processes of **absorption** (described in Chapter 3) **electrons** are removed from **atoms** within the irradiated material. After losing a negative particle, an atom is no longer electrical neutral: it becomes a positively charged **ion**. But then, unless acted on by a force that keeps them apart, the positive ion and negative ion (electron) normally recombine, releasing the absorbed energy that first separated them.

The ion creation/recombination sequence can be complex and significant. Some cells escape damage when X-rays ionise their atoms but others are affected in a way that leads to biological harm, possibly irreversible, with eventual, fatal consequences. For this reason, X-rays are used for diagnostic imaging *only if the potential benefits* – diagnosis or confirmation of a suspected medical condition, leading to early, correct treatment – *are confidently expected to outweigh any potential detriment or risk to the patient's well-being.*

fact that electricity, gas and petrol are forms of energy purchased for the sole purpose of using them in other forms. Gas is converted into heat and light; petrol is converted into kinetic energy (movement of a vehicle); and electricity is additionally convertible into sound and a whole range of electronic phenomena.

Kinetic energy is possessed by a body while in motion.
Potential energy is possessed by a body *within a field* – gravitational, electrical, magnetic, etc.

Absorption

Absorption is defined as *the transfer of energy from an X-ray beam to any object in its path*. Transferral is accompanied by conversion: irradiated objects do not contain X-rays; the radiant energy usually becomes kinetic or potential energy but there can be other outcomes. For example, when X-ray energy is absorbed by a phosphor, fluorescence occurs: conversion into visible light or ultraviolet radiation.

Atoms, electrons and ions

All matter is composed of elements – oxygen, hydrogen, carbon, iron, etc. The smallest (unit) particle of an element that retains its characteristics is an atom (Figure 1.2). For the purposes of understanding most X-ray processes, a very simple model of atomic structure is sufficient. The atom can be imagined as having a 'planetary' form with a central, positively-charged nucleus, around which negatively-charged electrons travel, in orbits. Orbiting electrons are held (by positive/negative attraction) at fixed, radial distances, in 'shells'.

An atom is electrically neutral: it contains equal numbers of positive charges (protons, within the nucleus) and negative charges (electrons arranged in the shells). Removal of a charge destroys the balance: it converts the atom into an ion. This process is termed *ionisation*. So, when the atom loses an electron, it becomes a positively-charged ion. The freed electron is a negative ion. Molecules (bonded groups of atoms) can be significantly changed by ionisation.

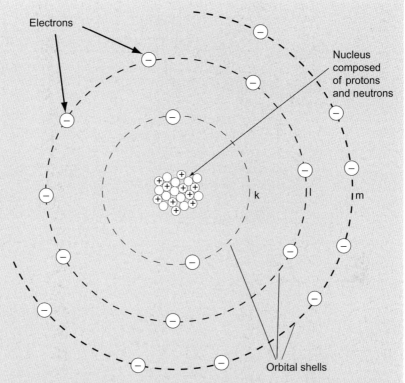

Figure 1.2 Simplified model of an atom. By mutual attraction, the positively-charged protons in the nucleus hold an equal number of negatively-charged electrons in orbit, in their shells – energy levels at fixed distances from the nucleus. The shells are conventionally labelled k, l, m, etc. A maximum is set for the number of electrons each shell can hold. The neutrons (no charge) maintain the stability of the nucleus: they prevent the protons, despite their 'like' charges, from being separated by mutual repulsion.

An advantage and a disadvantage

X-rays are invisible, silent and altogether undetectable by any of the human senses. It can be argued that this lack of detectable properties is an advantage: it can helpfully reduce the anxiety of a nervous patient. But it can also be regarded as a disadvantage: many of those who pioneered research into X-radiation and its application were unaware of its dangers. Today, warnings to exclude members of the public from areas of high X-ray intensity require physical reinforcement.

Occupational and medical exposure

Radiation protection must be extended to every person who is or may be exposed to ionising radiation. But a clear distinction must be made between

- *medical* exposure of a patient who receives the benefit of diagnostic information, which outweighs and justifies the potential risk, and
- *occupational* exposure of a member of staff, which is accidental and can bring no benefit of any kind.

What about protection of persons who are neither patients nor staff?

A limited number of persons fall into a category that lies between medical and occupational exposure. These are principally people who, having been fully informed about the potential risks, consent to attend close to a patient during the course of an X-ray examination, in a support role. For example, parents may stay with nervous children, and a friend or relative may offer a steadying hand to a frail or elderly patient.

These persons must be equipped with protection (e.g. a lead rubber apron) and instructed how risks can be minimised. Such an event – even though it may involve an individual only once – must be fully documented.

Phosphors and luminescence

Phosphors are chemicals that have the property of absorbing radiant energy and re-emitting it in a changed (lower energy) form. Emission of light from a phosphor, which may be either immediate or delayed until after a storage period, is termed *luminescence*

Fluorescence

This term describes *immediate* luminescence. An example occurs when an intensifying screen is exposed to X-rays. Energy is emitted

The risk of biological harm also lies behind the complex legislation that protects health-care staff and members of the general public (not patients). If accidentally exposed to radiation hazards, these persons cannot possibly receive any benefit from the experience.

Ionisation is rightly regarded as a dangerous feature of exposure to X-rays. But it must be noted that other effects of ionisation, where living cells are *not* involved, are essential to image formation. These include stimulation of luminescent materials, photographic effect and ionisation of gas and matter.

Stimulation of luminescent materials

If inanimate and stable materials are exposed to X-rays, ionisation is normally followed simply by recombination: negative and positive ions rejoin, restoring atoms to their previous state. But when the separation/recombination sequence happens within some specialised chemicals, termed **phosphors**, the phenomenon of **luminescence** occurs. Phosphors absorb energy from the X-ray beam then re-emit it in the form of ultraviolet rays and visible light. **Fluorescence** (*immediate* re-emission) is widely used in X-ray imaging: for example, through the action of **intensifying screens**. **Phosphorescence** (*delayed* re-emission) is used in **dosimetry** and in some methods of digital imaging.

Photographic effect

Under special conditions, ionisation of inanimate matter can also produce irreversible effects. This happens when a photographic film is exposed. Sensitive film emulsions contain unstable crystals of silver salts that achieve stability by absorbing energy. First, exposure to electromagnetic radiation energy causes partial conversion to silver. This occurs on a microscopically small scale but sufficiently to allow successful completion (the second stage) when the film is chemically developed. Photographic emulsions are sensitive to direct X-ray exposure but also to visible light and ultraviolet rays emitted from phosphors, in response to X-ray stimulation (absorption).

Ionisation of gas and matter

Ionisation within a precisely measured volume of gas, in an 'ionisation chamber', can be used as a reliable method of measuring X-radiation, bringing accuracy to radiographic exposures.

during the exposure in the form of ultraviolet radiation and visible light.

Intensifying screens

These are plastic sheets, of sizes identical to X-ray films, used to sandwich a film during its exposure to X-rays, within a lightproof cassette. One surface of a screen is coated with a layer containing phosphor crystals, which fluoresce when they absorb X-ray energy, considerably increasing the energy that the film receives from X-rays alone.

Phosphorescence

This is *delayed* emission of energy from a phosphor. An example is the light emitted from a 'luminous' warning sign that absorbs light energy during the day and remains visible during hours of darkness.

Dosimetry

The science of measuring X-ray doses and interpreting their significance.

Projection

This term is used to describe both the path through the patient's body along which an X-ray beam is directed, and the image it produces.

Image receptor

The X-ray beam emerging from the patient's body carries information about the exposed object, based on its various areas of radiopacity or radiolucency. In its radiation form, this information is invisible. The image receptor is the device used to convert the radiation pattern into a visible image.

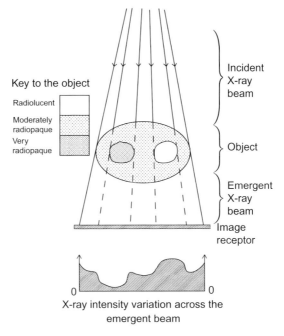

Key to the object

Radiolucent

Moderately radiopaque

Very radiopaque

Incident X-ray beam

Object

Emergent X-ray beam

Image receptor

X-ray intensity variation across the emergent beam

Figure 1.3 Formation of the emergent X-ray beam. Unlike the uniform intensity of the incident X-ray beam, the emergent beam comprises a variety of intensities, due to the object's radiopacities, radiolucencies, and variations in thickness (i.e. the dimension along which the photons travel). The intensities form an invisible energy pattern – a 'radiation image' – conveying information about the object that becomes visible after absorption by the image receptor and processing.

Ionisation due to X-ray exposure can also usefully occur in semiconductors and in other electronic devices, including the 'direct capture' image receptors used in the production of digital X-ray images.

The principles of X-ray image formation

X-ray images are formed by **projection**: a beam of X-rays is projected through the object under examination, casting its shadows on to an **image receptor** (Figure 1.3).

If a single, stationary image is required, the long-established method involves recording it on a sheet of photographic film. After exposure, the film is chemically processed, to become a **radiograph**. Alternatively, in a **computed** or **digital radiography** system, a radiation-sensitive phosphor plate is used. The collected data are electronically processed and displayed as an image on a computer monitor.

Radiograph

The familiar plastic sheets, bearing black and white images, are popularly referred to as 'X-rays'. But among professionals concerned with medical imaging, who understand that X-rays are invisible, the term *radiograph* – an image created by radiation – prevents ambiguity.

Computed and digital radiography

Both terms describe a radiographic imaging system where information about X-ray attenuation and transmission through an object is formed or converted into digital data, from which a computer constructs a visible image. *Computed* radiography involves radiation-sensitive phosphor plates that are exposed (in a similar fashion to films) then scanned, to extract the collected data. Images are constructed from the data, after processing by a computer. *Digital* radiography systems, though more complex and expensive, are quicker; their image input devices directly 'capture' data from the X-ray beam.

Dynamic images

In contrast to a stationary image, dynamic images show movement (functioning) of the patient's body 'in real time'. They are essential for obtaining diagnostic information in situations where a static image is inadequate – e.g. during ultrasound investigations and X-ray fluoroscopy.

Fluoroscopy

This is the procedure used to form a dynamic X-ray image. It is used (instead of stationary, radiographic images) when the patient's body needs to be 'watched' rather than simply 'seen', where immediate feedback to the operator is essential for guiding surgical or other interventional procedures. It can also find a use as a preliminary aid to radiographic positioning, where precision is being threatened by structural abnormalities.

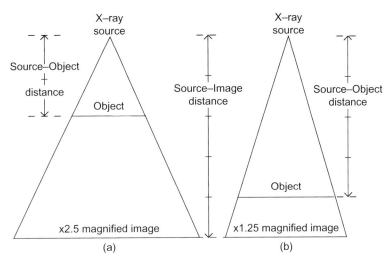

Figure 1.4 X-ray image magnification. The X-ray beam's divergence unavoidably produces an image larger than the object. The *ratio between *source–image distance* and *source–object distance* forms the **magnification factor**. Provided these distances are known, true linear dimensions of an object (e.g. width or length) can be calculated by applying the magnification factor inversely to dimensions measured on the image. [Radiographic techniques favour restricting magnification because, though its cause is different, the same distances affect geometric unsharpness. (*In these examples, the distance ratios are: (a) 5:2 and (b) 5:4.)]

Where a **dynamic image** is required, so that the object's motion can be watched, a fluorescent screen is normally used, fronting an electronic/optical viewing system. This procedure is known as **fluoroscopy**.

Magnification

All shadows formed by the action of a divergent X-ray beam are larger than the objects they represent. This is similar to the magnification of shadows cast by visible light from a small, **discrete** source, such as a light bulb. The effects on X-ray and visible light shadows of changing the distances are also similar: as an object is separated more widely from its shadow, magnification increases (Figure 1.4).

Lack of the third dimension

Even when they fall on curved or irregular surfaces, shadows cast by sunlight or a light bulb only have two dimensions: they show an

What is 'screening'?

Within an Imaging Department, 'screening' is the popular term for 'fluoroscopy'. Its use dates back to times when the fluorescent image was actually formed on a simple, phosphor-coated screen, which had to be observed in a totally darkened room. This term is deep-rooted but its users should be aware that, just as when 'X-ray' is used instead of 'radiograph', there is a risk of ambiguity: 'screening' is a term in its own right, indicating procedures carried out to confirm or exclude a specified condition or disease.

Magnification

All projected X-ray images are larger than the objects they represent. The cause is the X-ray beam's divergence. The amount of magnification depends on the separation between an object and the plane where its image is formed: as separation increases, the image becomes larger.

An image's diagnostic information is normally unaffected by magnification, because images are *expected to be* slightly larger than life-size, and in some circumstances, magnification can make the image easier to interpret. If accurate measurement of the object is required, a correction factor can be calculated.

Discrete

This term is used, particularly in scientific texts, to indicate that something is distinct, with definable boundaries. For example, a light bulb is a discrete light source; a cloudy sky is not. X-ray photons are often described as 'discrete' – meaning that each represents a distinct, limited quantity of radiant energy. (This word should not be confused with 'discreet' – meaning tactful, designed to avoid embarrassment.)

Lack of the third dimension

Binocular vision tends to be taken for granted. So everyone new to viewing X-ray images needs to become aware that projections from a single X-ray source cannot show an object's 'depth'.

One

object's width and height but they cannot demonstrate its depth. X-ray shadows are similarly restricted, leading to X-ray image *distortion* and *superimposition*.

Distortion

If incorrectly projected, an X-ray image can misrepresent the object's shape. It can be **foreshortened** or **elongated**, depending on the angle of the object in relation to (i) the X-ray beam and (ii) the plane of the image receptor (Figure 1.5). Distorted X-ray images offer only limited diagnostic information, and may even be deceptive.

Superimposition

When two or more structures are lined up along the path of a beam of light or X-rays, their shadows are superimposed. If the structures are of comparable, limited radiopacity, their separate images may combine, with confusing results. If one of the structures is larger or more radiopaque, it can obscure the other(s) completely (Figure 1.6).

Standardised projections

To minimise image distortion:

▪ the X-ray beam should be directed at right angles towards the object plane;
▪ the image receptor should be positioned parallel to the object plane.

It can be difficult to meet this theoretical ideal completely, because few structures within the human body have single, identifiable 'planes', and within complex regions such as the thorax and abdomen, many 'objects' are crowded together, at various angles. So, it is impossible for most X-ray images totally to escape the problems posed by distortion and by superimposition.

'*Two projections, mutually at right angles*' can resolve some difficulties, but not all: sometimes, anatomical restrictions intervene; and when extra projections are considered, their benefits must be weighed against the risks of further exposure.

A camera only has one lens. Why aren't photographs also limited to two dimensions?

In fact, they are. But a skilled photographer can use light and shade and perspective to suggest 'depth'. Our perceptions of photographs are also influenced by familiarity and simple logic.

Aren't foreshortening and elongation opposites? – Can't they cancel each other out?

No, because their causes are different. Foreshortening occurs when the X-ray beam being projected through the object meets the object plane at an oblique angle. Elongation occurs *after* the X-ray beam has passed through the object. It can further distort the *already formed* pattern of X-ray shadows before it reaches the image receptor, but it cannot correctly rearrange them.

Projection terminology

Apart from a few that are named after the persons credited with inventing them, projections are described according to the path of the X-ray beam through the object.

- **Anteroposterior (AP)** projections are produced when the X-ray beam enters the object's anterior surface and leaves through its posterior surface 'from front to back'. (The normal anatomical position indicates whether a surface is anterior or posterior.)
- **Postero-anterior (PA)** projections involve a reverse situation: the X-ray beam travels 'from the back to the front'.
- **Lateral** projections, taken 'from the side', are used to complement AP and/or PA projections by presenting information about the third dimension, which they have failed to show

Occasionally, information about this third dimension is better provided by an *inferosuperior* or a *supero-inferior* projection, with the beam passing along or parallel to the body's axis. There are other instances where a projection is named anatomically, according to the entry and exit surfaces. A *dorsiplantar* projection of the foot is an example.

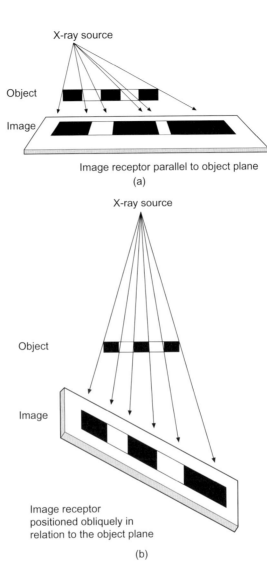

Image receptor parallel to object plane

(a)

Image receptor
positioned obliquely in
relation to the object plane

(b)

Figure 1.5 X-ray image distortion (a) X-rays approaching the object plane at approximately 90 degrees produce a relatively undistorted image, provided that the image receptor is positioned parallel to the object plane. But oblique rays tend to foreshorten the image – shown in this example as a loss of the equal spacing between the object's 'radiopaque' and 'radiolucent' parts; as obliquity increases, the radiopaque blocks cast larger shadows, while the radiolucent spaces become narrower. (b) Distortion tends to be avoided by centring the X-ray beam at right angles to the object's principal plane. This benefit is carried by the emergent beam – but it can only become a feature of the visible image if the image receptor is positioned parallel to the object plane. Oblique positioning creates varied magnification across the image: as the gap widens (i.e. as the ratio reduces between *source–object* and *object–image* distances) magnification increases, elongating the image – seen in this example as enlargement, from left to right, in the shadows of *both* 'radiopaque' and 'radiolucent' parts.

One

Does it matter whether a projection is anteroposterior or postero-anterior?

If the (anatomical) object is both narrow and shallow, *AP* and *PA* projections may be virtually identical. But this similarity can't be achieved with larger objects, because the X-rays' divergence produces a spread of shadows, which depends on the beam's direction. The choice between an *AP* or a *PA* projection may be guided by one or more of the following:

- the effects of beam divergence: *is the object 'opened up' with reduced superimposition and distortion, or the reverse?*
- situation of the area of particular interest: *is it located anteriorly or posteriorly?* If closer to the image receptor, geometric unsharpness will tend to be reduced.
- the shape of the object: *is there a curvature that matches the divergence of the X-ray beam – or conflicts with it, increasing superimposition and distortion?*
- the patient's condition, particularly following trauma: *will the patient be safer if the normal projection, on this occasion, is reversed to avoid causing pain or aggravation of the condition?*
- the need for immobilisation: *will the patient find a modified technique easier and more comfortable?*
- radiation protection: *are there some particularly radiosensitive structures that can be partially shielded if they are positioned nearer to the image receptor than to the X-ray tube?*

The importance of symmetry

Interpretation of AP and PA projections taken when the beam's central ray passes along the body's median plane is critically assisted by the normal symmetry of the skeleton: left mirrors right. Following trauma, for example, an unaffected side can act as a 'control' against which the extent of damage to the affected side can be judged. This possibility reinforces the need for careful positioning – excluding rotation – to preserve symmetry and potentially increase diagnostic information.

One

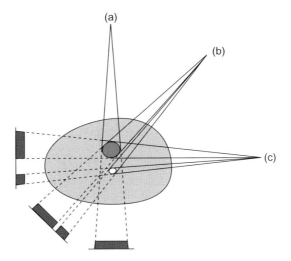

Figure 1.6 Superimposition. A small, radiolucent structure aligned within the path of the X-ray beam, behind a larger, radiopaque structure (a) fails to appear in the projected image. Angulation of the X-ray beam, either obliquely (b) or at right angles (c) to the axis of alignment, separates the shadows and shows the structures independently.

To support the principle of maximising diagnostic information, while minimising radiation hazards, a system of standardised projections has evolved within X-ray imaging. This aims to prevent or reduce the misrepresentations and illusions that can arise from the two-dimensional nature of X-ray images.

There are three factors involved.

Positioning of the patient

The positioning procedure should be simple enough to be followed accurately and identically, time after time. Supine, prone and erect (or seated) positions are most common but the patient can also be rotated or otherwise repositioned through 90 degrees or some other measurable, oblique angle.

Direction and centring of the X-ray beam

The X-ray beam's approach to the object is normally specified in relation to anatomical landmarks. The body's median plane is prominent in techniques involving the head, neck, thorax, abdomen and pelvis; techniques for the limbs rely strongly on anatomical surface markings.

Projections and positions

Radiographic projections are not absolutely dependent on the patient's position, provided that their relationship to the X-ray beam and the image receptor is correct. A lateral projection of the cervical vertebrae, for instance, may be exposed with the patient either upright or lying supine. So there is a distinction between projections and positions. Sometimes, the orientation of the X-ray beam will be standardised – for instance, a horizontal beam is necessary for demonstrating a fluid/gas interface (a 'fluid level').

There will often be a preferred patient position – for example, in the case of the lateral projection of the cervical vertebrae, an upright position allows the force of gravity to reduce superimposition of the patient's shoulders on the lower vertebrae. But it is a hallmark of experience to achieve a standard projection (image) despite restriction of the patient to an unfavourable, non-standard position.

Integrated X-ray equipment and the isocentric principle

The accuracy of the X-ray tube, patient and image receptor positioning may depend on the versatility of the X-ray equipment. Despite being safe and accurate, some older units lack convenience and comfort; patients have to be positioned 'to fit the equipment', with all the awkwardness that it entails. Modern equipment design has favoured a permanently linked and centred X-ray tube and image receptor to 'fit around the patient'. This is especially valuable if the patient is injured or unconscious, but in all cases, the correct relationship between X-ray tube, object and image receptor is easier to obtain, X-ray beam collimation can be very precise – and both image quality and radiation protection increase. This is especially so when both X-ray tube and image receptor are mounted on an assembly that can be rotated about a common axis, positioned to coincide with the centre of the object: the *isocentric* principle.

Point source

A slide or ciné projector can form a sharp image on a distant screen, many hundreds of times larger than the original film frame, because its optical system focuses light to act as if it comes from an infinitely small *point source*. Unfortunately, X-rays cannot be focused; lenses

One

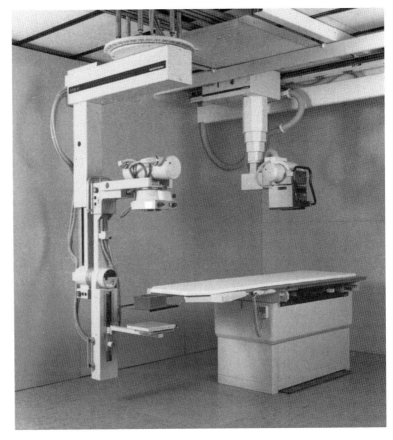

Figure 1.7 Isocentric and conventional X-ray equipment. Isocentric equipment (on the left) has an X-ray tube linked and centred to the image receptor, allowing it to be correctly positioned with ease *around the patient*, producing image projections from any angle. This flexibility is particularly valuable for examinations of the limbs and their principal joints, and the skull. It potentially reduces image distortion, and minimises the need for awkward positioning of the patient. Conventional equipment (on the right) is less versatile: it tends to require the patient to be positioned to suit its own restricted range of angulations (by courtesy of Siemens Medical plc).

Positioning of the image receptor

This is often simply horizontal or vertical, especially when basic, standard X-ray equipment is used. Other, more specialised equipment, including units based on the **isocentric** principle (Figure 1.7), allow the image receptor plane to be angled to suit an individual patient, reducing image distortion and improving the patient's comfort.

and mirrors placed in the path of an X-ray beam simply absorb some of its energy. So, as far as X-ray imaging is concerned, a *point source* remains a theoretical, rather than a practical concept.

Penumbra

This is the zone of partial shadow that surrounds true, full shadow, when formed by light or X-rays emanating from a source of measurable proportions – that is, not a 'point source'.

Geometric unsharpness

This may be seen on a radiographic image: the visible form of X-ray penumbra. Its magnitude is controlled by the size of the X-ray tube's focal spot and by the ratio between the *focus–object* and *object–image receptor* distances.

Resolution

This term indicates a system's capacity to detect and/or record 'detail'. It is proportional to the smallness of the component parts within its detection/recording area. The resolution of the eye's retina depends on the size and healthy state of its component cells; digital image resolution is proportional to the number of picture elements ('pixels') arrayed within its detection area. The resolution of photographic film is limited by the size and shape of the sensitive crystals in its emulsion, and the thickness of the emulsion layer. Intensifying screens similarly depend on the characteristics of their phosphor layers.

Communication, co-operation and immobilisation

The key to preventing movement unsharpness often lies in making the patient comfortable, and communicating the simple requirement, when the moment comes, to keep still. Most patients are very pleased to co-operate. If respiration is involved, a short rehearsal can be helpful. If extra support is needed, it should be offered gently, with encouragement.

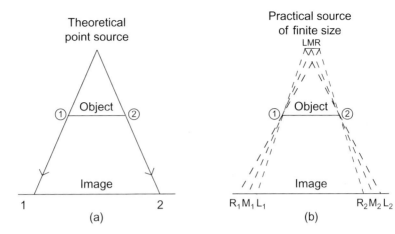

Figure 1.8 The cause of geometric unsharpness. (a) The ideal, theoretical use of a 'point source' of X-rays would produce an absolutely sharp image. (b) The practical source has small but measurable dimensions. It acts as a tight cluster of sources, each producing a separate shadow of the object, from its left-hand edge (L), through the middle (M), across to the right-hand edge (R). The shadows are grouped together and although they overlap in the centre, there is incomplete shadowing – the X-ray penumbra – at the margins, forming geometric unsharpness on the visible image.

Image unsharpness

Whatever its cause, unsharpness can reduce the diagnostic information that an X-ray image offers, so it must be eliminated whenever possible. There are three potential causes.

Geometric unsharpness

Some shadows formed by visible light have sharply defined outlines, while others are indistinct. Sharpness, or the lack of it, can be traced to (a) the size of the light source, and (b) the ratio between the distances: from the light source to the object producing the shadow, and from the object to the plane where the shadow is cast.

A light source that is infinitely small, termed a **point source**, will produce sharp shadows, whatever distances are involved. But when the source has a measurable size, shadows tend to be surrounded by a zone of partial shadow, a **penumbra**, which blurs their edges (Figure 1.8).

With the aid of lenses and mirrors, projected visible light, whatever the actual size of its source, can appear and behave as if it comes from a point source. The circumstances surrounding X-ray

One

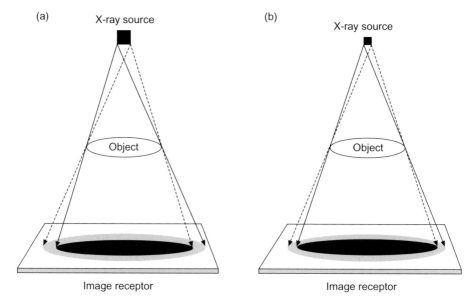

Figure 1.9 Factors affecting geometric unsharpness – 1: focal spot size. A dual-focus X-ray tube offers a choice of X-ray source sizes: (a) the penumbra formed by the larger, 'broad' focus spreads to form a degree of geometric unsharpness that may reduce the image's diagnostic value; (b) a change to the smaller, 'fine' focus restricts the penumbra's width, limiting geometric unsharpness.

image production are less encouraging. X-rays (a) cannot be produced from a point source, and (b) unlike visible light, cannot be focused. So, when X-ray shadows are formed, there is a penumbra, and images have an inherent **geometric unsharpness**. Its prime cause is the size of the X-ray source but it also depends on the ratio between the *source-to-object* and *object-to-image* distances (Figures 1.9 and 1.10).

Image receptor resolution

When invisible X-ray shadows are converted into visible X-ray images, further unsharpness may be introduced. Image receptors have a property known as **resolution**. This indicates how faithfully the fine detail carried within X-ray shadows is detected and displayed. Ideally, an image receptor's resolution is matched to the level of detail contained within a given X-ray shadow. If resolution exceeds this level, nothing is lost; but if resolution is too coarse, it can add to the image's unsharpness.

When conventional materials are used, the effect on a radiographic image of a film emulsion's resolution, and the (probably

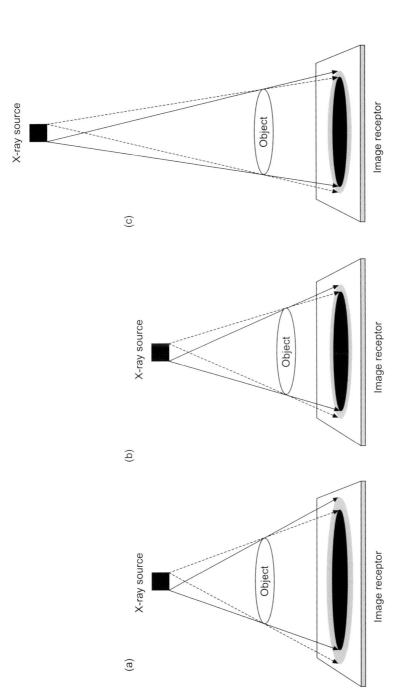

Figure 1.10 Factors affecting geometric unsharpness – 2: ratio between the *source (focus)–object* and *object–image* distances. The relatively large geometric unsharpness shown in (a) can usually be reduced by positioning the object closer to the image receptor – shown in (b). This shortens the *object–image* distance, at the same time lengthening the *source–object* distance, so increasing the ratio between them. If circumstances prevent the object being repositioned closer to the image receptor, a similar ratio increase may be achievable by repositioning the X-ray source further away from the object (c) – i.e. by increasing the *source–object* distance alone.

Radiolucent and radiopaque

A *radiolucent* structure allows X-rays to pass through it relatively easily. The term *radiopaque* describes a structure that tends to prevent the passage of X-rays. But practically all substances show a degree of both radiolucency and radiopacity. So these terms tend to be used relatively – to compare one structure with another.

The use of artificial contrast agents

Many structures within the body are not naturally visible on an X-ray image because they are too similar to their surroundings, in terms of their radiopacity or radiolucency. In some cases, a temporary change may be produced: a radiopaque contrast agent can be introduced into a blood vessel or body cavity, increasing its radiopacity. Alternatively, or additionally, a cavity can be filled with a gas that, because of its very low density, makes the structure temporarily radiolucent.

Artefacts

These are *accidental* inclusions within a radiographic image, potentially obscuring its diagnostic information, or suggesting false information by mimicking anatomical or pathological appearances. They can be caused at any stage during the exposure and processing of an image but are typically due to neglect of Quality Assurance protocols.

Identification of X-ray images

All X-ray images must carry permanent identification data because they are, in effect, medical documents. Potentially also, they have legal significance. Information must include the patient's identity, the date and time of the image, and the hospital or clinic where the image was exposed.

more significant) influence of intensifying screens, is normally termed photographic unsharpness.

Movement unsharpness

Both radiographic (stationary, single) and fluoroscopic images can be affected by geometric unsharpness and the image receptor's resolution. Fluoroscopy is a procedure used specifically for watching movement: respiration, peristalsis, etc.; but in the production of a stationary, radiographic image, *movement can cause unsharpness*. This can be avoided by temporarily keeping the object motionless, and by use of a short exposure time.

Image contrast

When an object is positioned in the path of an X-ray beam, *each of its internal parts* potentially casts its own shadow. Superimposed one upon another, these together form a composite X-ray image. Structures that allow X-rays to pass through them with relative ease are termed **radiolucent.** Others, offering more resistance to the passage of X-rays, are said to be **radiopaque**. So an X-ray image represents a whole object according to the relative radiopacity or radiolucency of its component parts.

To be visible within an X-ray image, a particular part of an object must, in some way, be distinct. A radiopaque structure *surrounded by others of equal radiopacity* will tend not to be shown. Similarly, a radiolucent area will be difficult to identify *if adjacent areas are equally radiolucent*. But an individual part, whether radiolucent or radiopaque, *will* be shown within a composite X-ray image, if it *contrasts with its surroundings*.

Many factors affect an X-ray image's contrast. Composition of the object is of primary importance but the list also includes:

▓   the parameters of the X-ray beam (discussed in Chapter 2),
▓   the interactions that occur when the beam passes through the object (Chapter 3), and
▓   the processes by which image contrast becomes visible (Chapter 4).

Summary of criteria for assessing an X-ray image

(a)   X-ray images should be free from avoidable distortion and superimposition.

Benefit versus risk: A consideration throughout health care

Weighing of *benefits* against *risks* is not confined to the requesting of diagnostic X-ray examinations; surgical procedures and the prescription of drugs also present potential complications or side-effects. In both these cases, risks must be weighed against the benefits of a potential cure.

(b) Geometric features of the beam should be controlled, to minimise image unsharpness.

(c) The image receptor's resolution should be fine enough to avoid adding to an image's unsharpness.

(d) No movement should be permitted during the exposure of (stationary image) radiographs.

(e) Images must have sufficient contrast to show the required structures of interest within the object.

In addition:

(f) An image must include the whole of the anatomical area needed for a complete diagnosis but (to confirm appropriate radiation protection) must not be significantly larger than required.

(g) An image must be free from any **artefacts** (blemishes) that could reduce its diagnostic value.

(h) All images must incorporate clear **identification data**, confirming at least the patient's identity, and the date, time and place of the examination.

The importance of justification

High standards are important because poor images are unlikely to have much diagnostic value. But image quality must never be pursued *for its own sake*; improvements achieved at the expense of the patient's physical and radiation safety, which *bring no increase in diagnostic benefit*, are unjustifiable. The *benefit versus risk* relationship requires continuous attention: all decisions that result in exposure of the patient to X-rays, not only when an examination is requested and assessed but during the examination itself, must be justified.

One

Chapter 2
Formation of the incident beam

Introduction

The range of X-ray examinations is so wide (from extremities to the abdomen) and patients are so varied (from babies to adults) that almost every image requires its own selected X-ray exposure, different from the last – and probably the next. *There is no single, multipurpose X-ray beam.*

With an increasing degree of automation, modern X-ray equipment quickly and easily sets the correct conditions for most exposures; but a full understanding of X-ray production and control is still necessary, for safe and accurate operation. This is particularly so when modifications to routine practice are required, to cope with particular or unusual circumstances.

X-ray production

The essential equipment comprises a **generator** and a **tube**, which together convert an input of electrical energy into an output of X-ray energy (Figure 2.1). This involves a sequence of stages, crucially including production of a stream of **electrons** travelling at high speed, and conversion of their **kinetic** energy into X-ray **photons**. In detail, these stages are achieved as follows.

Production of free electrons

An X-ray tube comprises two main parts: a central **insert** within an oil-filled **housing** (Figure 2.2). The insert takes the form of an

X-ray generator

This is the equipment unit that supplies the specialised electrical voltages required by the X-ray tube, according to the selection of exposure factors, etc., at its control panel. A generator contains multiple compensation and control circuits that enable it to function accurately, reliably and safely.

X-ray tube

This is the electrical device where a sequence of energy conversions takes place, leading to the production of X-rays. It requires voltage supplies of differing values so it cannot simply be connected to 'the mains'. Instead, it draws its supplies from an X-ray generator.

Electrons

The negatively-charged particles that orbit the nucleus of an atom, held in discrete shells at fixed, radial distances by the positive, attractive force of the nucleus.

Kinetic energy

Energy possessed by a body while in motion.
The term *kinetic* can also be regarded as indicating a *group* of energy forms, including *electrical energy* (electric charge in linear motion) and *heat* (atoms and molecules in vibrational motion).

X-ray photon

Also known as a *quantum*, a photon is produced by an energy-conversion interaction within an X-ray tube. It is a discrete quantity of X-ray energy but not a fixed-value unit; there are high-energy photons and low-energy photons.

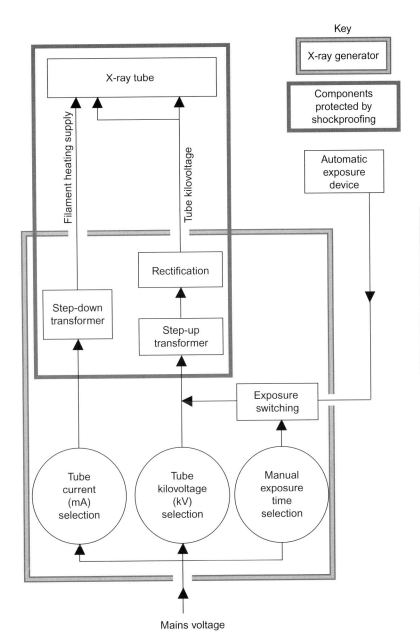

Figure 2.1 Equipment for X-ray production. This schematic plan shows the principal components of an X-ray generator, responsible for the specialised energy supplies required by an X-ray tube.

X-ray tube insert

This is the inner part of an X-ray tube. It comprises an evacuated envelope, usually made of glass, into which are sealed the tube's anode and cathode. Closely fitted outside the envelope, in the region of the anode rotor, is the electrical assembly (the 'stator windings') responsible for making the anode rotate.

X-ray tube housing

This is the metallic container, usually cylindrical, forming the outer part of an X-ray tube, surrounding and protecting the tube insert. Its sealed cavity is filled with oil that provides electrical insulation for the internal wiring. The oil also plays a part in cooling the tube, convecting heat from the insert to the wall of the housing.

A radiolucent opening, the window or port, allows X-rays to emerge, to form the 'useful beam'. But because X-rays are emitted from the face of the target in all directions (not just towards the window) most of the housing is lined with sheet lead, moulded to fit the contours of its walls.

As the tube's temperature rises, the oil expands. To prevent pressure from building up within the cavity, part of the housing wall is formed by a flexible diaphragm that moves in and out, allowing the oil's volume safely to expand and contract.

Envelope

This is the wall of the insert, usually made of heat-resistant ('ovenware') glass: radiolucent, inert, strong and an electrical insulator. In some specialised cases, the envelope may be made of metal, with ceramic insulation of its electrical terminals.

Cathode

This is the X-ray tube's electrode connected to the high *negative* potential (kilovoltage) produced by the generator. It houses two* focusing cups, each surrounding a linear spiral filament (*because, with few exceptions, diagnostic X-ray tubes are 'dual-focus').

Anode

This is the X-ray tube's electrode that operates at a high *positive* potential, (kilovoltage) produced by the generator. In most diagnostic X-ray tubes, the anode comprises a *disc*, mounted on a short, narrow *stem*, arising from a cylindrical *rotor*. This assembly rotates on an axial support, when receiving energy from the tube's stator windings.

Filament

This is a length of thin, uninsulated tungsten wire, wound into a linear spiral. When a current flows through it, increased atomic vibration raises its temperature, until it becomes incandescent, like a light bulb's filament. It then releases electrons, by the process of thermionic emission. Filament temperature is controlled by the tube current (mA) selector.

A dual-focus diagnostic X-ray tube has two separate filaments, of different sizes. Heating of one or the other ('broad' or 'fine') is selected at the generator's control panel. The selected option changes the area on the anode where X-ray production takes place – so the control is actually termed the 'focal spot (or focus) selector'.

Tungsten as a filament material

Tungsten is widely used in equipment operating at high temperatures because it has the highest melting point of any metallic element (3 300°C) and it has a relatively low vaporisation rate, i.e. it changes from solid into vapour only slowly, even at high temperatures.

Filaments are made of tungsten because of these properties, but also because it can be drawn out into a fine wire (it is described as 'ductile') which is strong, retaining its shape even when white-hot. Tungsten is a ready, controllable emitter of electrons, requiring only a relatively low electrical energy supply.

Current

This term describes the flow of electric charge that occurs through a conductor in response to a voltage (potential difference) applied across it. It is measured as a *rate of flow* – i.e. as the quantity of charge passing a given point, per unit time.

The unit of current is the ampere (symbol, A). 1 ampere indicates a rate of flow of *1 coulomb of electric charge per second*.

Voltage (potential difference)

An electrical potential difference – commonly referred to as a *voltage* – across a conductor (when part of a circuit) causes the electrons within it to move and form a current. The unit used to measure electrical potential (and potential difference) is the volt (symbol, V), which defines the amount of energy possessed by unit charge: *1 joule per coulomb*.

Thermionic emission

This is the emission of electrons from a heated filament.

If a filament is heated for a long time, doesn't it lose all its electrons?

No. When the X-ray tube's filament is at a low temperature, *between* exposures, the emission of electrons (because they are negative) makes the filament positive, so it continuously re-attracts them. A state of equilibrium develops; the filament is surrounded by an electron cloud or 'space charge' of a size in proportion to the rate of heating (supply of energy).

During exposures, when the filament temperature is raised and the emission rate is high, the electrons that travel across to the anode are continuously followed (replaced) by other electrons, flowing around the whole of the high-voltage circuit, forming the X-ray tube current.

Kilovoltage

This is the term used to describe the potential difference applied across an X-ray tube (between anode and cathode) because it is measured in kilovolts (symbol kV). One kilovolt is one thousand volts.

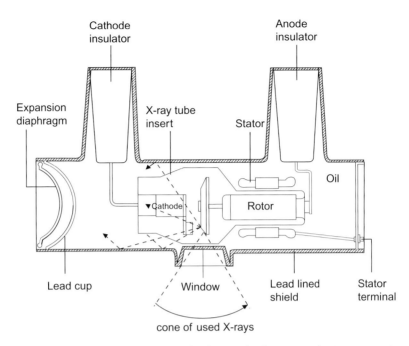

Figure 2.2 A rotating anode X-ray tube (longitudinal section). The insert containing the anode and cathode is held within a protecting shield or housing that ensures physical, electrical and radiation safety (by courtesy of IGE Medical Systems).

envelope containing two electrodes: the **cathode** and **anode**. The cathode incorporates a **filament**, a small coil of **tungsten** wire, heated by a **current**, in response to a low **voltage**, supplied by the generator.

As the current flows, its electrons transfer some of their kinetic energy to the filament's atoms, making them vibrate more vigorously. This extra vibration raises the filament's temperature: it glows brightly, emitting heat and light. At the same time, by the process of **thermionic emission**, *it emits free electrons*.

The emitted electrons' acquisition of kinetic energy

Emission from the filament alone gives the electrons very little kinetic energy. To acquire more, they require a much stronger influence. This is provided when the X-ray generator's 'exposure' button is pressed, connecting a **kilovoltage** (usually between 50 kV and 120 kV) across the X-ray tube: the cathode becomes very strongly negative, and the anode, a short distance away, very strongly positive. Immediately, electrons emitted from the filament are now

Scientific symbols – the importance of case

It is important that symbols for scientific units are written accurately, using the correct lower-case or upper-case (capital) letters – i.e. scientific symbols are *case-sensitive*. With only 26 letters available plus a few characters from the Greek alphabet, most letters have two roles to play. For example, the lower-case symbol 'k' represents the prefix kilo-, while an upper-case (capital) K indicates *kelvin*, the unit of absolute temperature.

The letter 'm' requires equal care because it is used to indicate two widely different orders of magnitude. The prefix indicating one-thousandth ($\times 10^{-3}$), 'milli-', is represented by the lower-case symbol 'm'. A capital 'M' indicates 'mega', meaning one million times, ($\times 10^{6}$).

Another point to remember is that scientific symbols are never modified to become plural: e.g. one hundred kilovolts is '100 kV' *not* '100 kVs'. The numerals alone are sufficient to indicate a plural quantity. (Used as a symbol, 's' indicates 'second' – the unit of time.)

Potential energy

This is possessed by a body *within a field* – gravitational, electrical, magnetic, etc.

Target

The target is the area of an X-ray tube's anode bombarded by the stream of electrons from the filament. The outcome of electron bombardment is X-ray production, so the target may also be defined as the radiation source. Other terms with virtually the same meaning are *focal spot* and *focus*.

Focusing cup

This is the hollowed-out recess or slot, in which an X-ray tube's filament is located. As part of the cathode, a focusing cup is at high negative potential, so it exerts a repelling force on electrons emitted from the filament (*like* repelling *like*). This action is essential in

within a strong electric field: they have a large measure of **potential energy**. Their response is to move across the X-ray tube, repelled by the cathode and attracted towards the anode. As they do so, their potential energy changes into kinetic energy until, by the time they reach the anode, the accelerating electrons are travelling at high speed.

The vacuum within the tube envelope enables these processes to take place freely: there are no gas molecules to suppress electron emission from the filament or to hinder their progress across to the anode.

Conversion of the electrons' kinetic energy into X-ray energy

The conditions for this conversion are partly provided within the previous stage. When leaving the cathode, instead of diverging as a result of mutual repulsion (which would be natural, because each carries a negative charge) the electrons are forced to converge and travel towards a specific part of the anode, the **target**. Convergence is achieved by the action of the **focusing cup** that borders the filament. It has a sharp outer rim where the negative electric field strength is intensified, shaping the emerging electrons into a narrowing stream.

The target is usually also made of **tungsten**. When the high-speed electrons bombard the target, most of them simply transfer their kinetic energy to the target's atoms. The atoms' rate of vibration increases, raising the target's temperature – so, the principal outcome is the production of heat. But a few of the electrons undergo more useful interactions – some or all of their kinetic energy is converted into X-ray energy, via one or other of two processes: production of braking radiation and production of characteristic X-radiation.

Production of braking radiation (bremsstrahlung)

This is the predominant process. It occurs when electrons travelling at high speed from the filament pass close enough to target atoms' **nuclei** to enter their electric fields (Figure 2.3). Here (positive acting on negative) they experience a force of attraction that *suddenly changes their direction of travel*. This sudden change converts some of the electrons' kinetic energy into X-ray energy. Each conversion incident produces an X-ray photon.

As it loses kinetic energy, an electron slows down – explaining the term for X-rays produced in this manner: 'braking radiation'

Two

shaping the electrons into a convergent stream that travels across to – *is focused on* – the tube's target.

'Opposites' and 'likes'

A general scientific rule, applying to *positive* and *negative* electrical charges and to *north* and *south* magnetic poles, states: 'opposites attract; likes repel'. The forces that keep similar charges or poles apart, or bring opposites together, are directly proportional to the product of their strengths and inversely proportional to the squared value of the distances that separate them.

Tungsten as a target material

The basic inefficiency of the X-ray production process (most electrons having their kinetic energy converted into heat) results in an X-ray tube's target reaching very high temperatures. Tungsten, with the highest melting point of any metallic element (3 300°C) is the first choice for target (focal track) construction. It is also favoured by tungsten's relatively low vaporisation rate (the change from solid into vapour that erodes its surface), which occurs only slowly, even at high temperatures. A further, very important reason is that tungsten's relatively high atomic number, 74, (i) enables the nuclei of the target atoms to exert a relatively strong pull on electrons (from the filament) during the process of bremsstrahlung production, and (ii) ensures a relatively high photon energy for its principal characteristic radiation.

Note: No connection should be inferred between tungsten's high atomic number and its high melting point.

Nuclei

This is the plural form of *nucleus*. Confusion often surrounds the plural forms of words imported into English from Latin and other foreign languages. To reduce the extra learning task, the simple addition of '-s' or '-es' to the singular form is normally acceptable, but where it would sound awkward (e.g. 'nucleusses') and when the correct plural form is in common use, these should be learned, too.

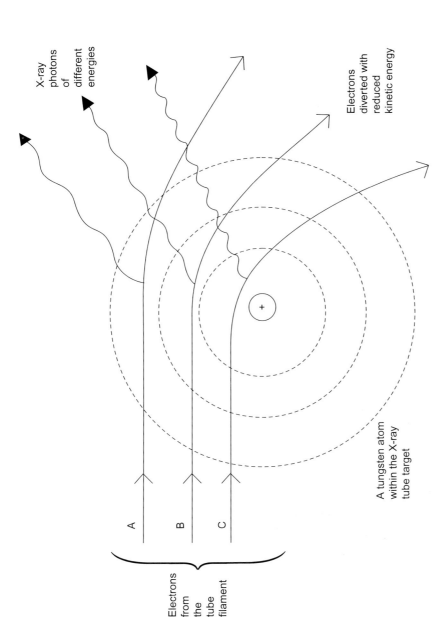

X-ray
photons
of
different
energies

Electrons
diverted with
reduced
kinetic energy

A tungsten atom
within the X-ray
tube target

Electrons
from
the
tube
filament

A

B

C

Figure 2.3 Production of X-ray bremsstrahlung. The electrons from the filament give three examples of the thousands of possible interactions occurring within the target during every X-ray exposure, that together produce a heterogeneous X-ray beam. The path of A brings it close enough to the atom's nucleus to experience a force of attraction, making it suddenly deviate, with conversion of some of its kinetic energy into an X-ray photon. Electron B passes closer to the nucleus and is more strongly affected; its deviation is sharper and the X-ray photon has more energy. The kinetic energy of electron C is converted even more efficiently; its path is closer to the atom's nucleus, deviation is the sharper and the outcome is a photon of higher energy than either A or B. Interactions such as A occur more often than B, which are more common than C.

Two

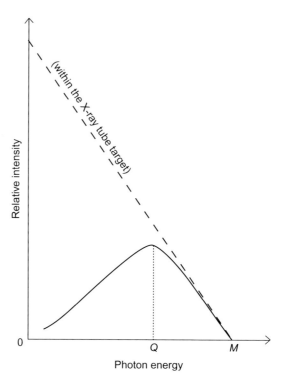

Figure 2.4 Bremsstrahlung: a typical continuous spectrum. This graph shows the relative intensities of bremsstrahlung photons, according to their energies. It illustrates (a) two important features of bremsstrahlung production: a range of photon energies is produced, forming a *continuous* spectrum; and fewer high-energy X-ray bremsstrahlung photons are produced than low-energy photons. It also shows (b) a disadvantage inherent in X-ray tube construction: since all photons originate *within the tube target*, they are subjected to significant absorption ('inherent filtration') along their paths from the target to the tube window.

The broken line represents X-ray production *within the tube target*. This has no practical significance but its negative slope confirms that fewer high-energy photons are produced than low-energy photons. The solid line represents photons emitted from the tube. It has a positive slope, showing that at energies rising from zero to Q, photons are emitted with increasing intensity, as penetration of the tube's inherent filtration becomes more successful, and a negative slope, due to the declining rate of higher-energy photon production, in the range Q to M (maximum). The highest intensity occurs at the junction between these two slopes, corresponding to the energy Q. This is the modal value, referred to as the beam's *quality*.

(or in German, the native language of Wilhelm Roentgen, the discoverer of X-rays, 'bremsstrahlung'). The vigour of an electron's reaction with a nucleus (and so, the percentage of its kinetic energy converted into X-ray energy) depends on the closeness of its path to the nucleus. Among the electrons as a whole, this distance varies, so, as Figure 2.4 shows, braking radiation photon energies span a

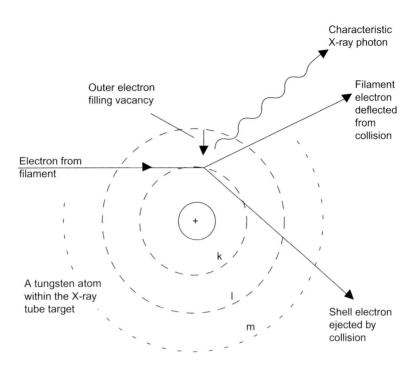

Figure 2.5 Production of characteristic X-ray photons. The kinetic energy of the filament electron is greater than the k shell binding energy. A collision with a k-shell electron is shown, creating a vacancy, filled in this case by an electron from the l shell. This incoming electron loses energy, equal to the difference between the binding energies of the two shells involved in the transition, which is converted into an X-ray photon.

range: from a calculable maximum value (assuming 100% conversion of an electron's kinetic energy) down to a small value at the lowest limit of measurement (when minimal energy is converted). *This energy range is significant.*

Production of characteristic X-radiation

This is the minor X-ray production process. It occurs when high-speed filament electrons collide with *electrons* orbiting a target atom's nucleus (Figure 2.5). Provided that a filament electron's kinetic energy is greater than the **binding energy** of the atom's electron, a collision results in removal of the electron from its shell, creating a vacancy. The atom's positive nucleus immediately attracts electrons from outer shells, to fill such vacancies. The outer electrons are in higher energy states, so the inward transitions cause them to lose energy. The energy lost during each transition is *converted into an X-ray photon.*

Significance of the bremsstrahlung energy range

Because of the way they are produced, bremsstrahlung photons have a range of energy values. So, although a tube kilovoltage is selected in proportion to the required beam penetration, it must be recognised that the beam contains a large proportion of photons of lower energy, including some that cannot reach beyond the object. These photons would present only 'risk' to the patient, with no compensating 'benefit'. The problem is addressed by the use of filtration.

Shell binding energy

Electrons orbiting the atom's nucleus are held within their shells by the force of attraction (positive acting on negative) exerted by the nucleus. This force acts more strongly on electrons nearer the nucleus. A shell's binding energy is defined as the energy required to remove one of its electrons. So, binding energies are higher for inner shells than for those further away from the nucleus.

Parameter

This term indicates a measurable, defining feature by which a given object or phenomenon may be distinguished from others that share the same fundamental properties. To illustrate, the maximum photon energy of an X-ray beam (due to the selected kilovoltage) is one of its *parameters*; straight-line propagation is a *property* it shares with other X-ray beams.

Heterogeneous

This term (not exclusive to X-ray imaging, or even to science) indicates a variety or mixture of values. Through the nature of its production, X-ray bremsstrahlung is heterogeneous: it comprises a range of photon energies, from an identifiable maximum, down to an indeterminate minimum. 'White' visible light, which contains a mixture of colours (wavelengths), is similarly heterogeneous.

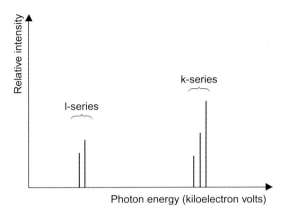

Figure 2.6 Line spectra. The identifiable photon energies of characteristic X-radiation, represented as line spectra, equal the differences between the shell binding energies, when vacancies are filled by electron transitions. The lines are grouped in 'series' according to the shells where vacancies are *filled*. From the nucleus outwards, shells are conventionally labelled k, l, m, etc. The number of lines in each series indicates the possible transitional jumps (fewer, for outer shells). The heights of the lines, showing relative intensities, indicate the amounts of energy produced in this way.

Unlike the range of unspecified braking radiation energies, characteristic X-ray photons have precise, predictable values (Figure 2.6). These equal *differences* between the binding energies of (i) the outer shells left by the electrons and (ii) the inner shells where they fill vacancies. Shell binding energies are unique to each element – which explains why X-ray photons produced by these vacancy-filling transitions are termed 'characteristic' X-rays.

X-ray beam control

X-ray beam parameters

Electrical factors selected at the generator's control panel and other equipment adjustments cannot influence the permanent properties of an X-ray beam (fixed velocity, straight-line propagation, etc.). But they have the important effect of establishing the X-ray beam's variable, measurable features: its **parameters**. Five will be considered – all within the control of the equipment's operator: maximum photon energy, beam quality, beam intensity, focal spot size and cross-sectional area (shape and size).

Types of spectrum

If a spectrum covers a range of consecutive values, it may be termed 'continuous'. X-ray bremsstrahlung, with an infinite number of varied photon energies forms a *continuous spectrum*.

Characteristic X-rays do not have consecutive values; their energies are fixed at intervals, related to the target material's shell binding energies. In graphic form, these are represented as *line spectra* (the plural form of 'spectrum') at identifiable points along the photon energy axis.

Mode/Modal

Mathematicians recognise three interpretations of the term 'average':

(1) The most familiar, the 'mean', is calculated by adding together the individual values under consideration, then dividing the sum by the number of individuals.

(2) The 'median' is the central value within the range.

(3) The 'mode' is an average derived from frequency or popularity: it identifies the *most commonly occurring* value within a group. The modal value is the most significant average measurement of the photon energies within the continuous X-ray spectrum. When an X-ray beam is represented in graphical form, the modal photon energy is identifiable by its coincidence with the highest relative intensity.

The kiloelectron volt

In mainstream science, energy is measured by use of the SI (Système International d'Unités) unit, the **joule** (symbol J). In X-ray imaging science, X-ray photon energies and electron binding energies are measured in kiloelectron volts (symbol keV). This specialised unit is used owing to its convenience.

An electron volt (symbol, eV) is defined as the energy gained by an electron when it is accelerated through a potential difference of 1 volt. So, a kiloelectron volt (keV) is the energy gained by an electron accelerated through a potential difference of 1 kilovolt. When an X-ray tube operates, this is fundamentally what happens:

Maximum photon energy

The selective nature of X-ray penetration implies that a beam passes easily through the radiolucent areas of an object but less easily through its radiopaque parts. Whether this actually occurs or not depends naturally on the object itself: in anatomical terms, its combination of 'soft tissue' (radiolucent) and skeletal (radiopaque) parts. But it also depends on the X-ray beam's maximum photon energy.

A maximum energy photon is the outcome of a single-event, 100% conversion of a filament electron's kinetic energy into X-ray energy (braking radiation). The selected kV gives electrons crossing the X-ray tube their kinetic energy. So, when X-ray beam parameters are being set for an exposure, kV selection is matched to the object's radiopacity. Otherwise, if the selected kV is too low (because the object's radiopacity has been underestimated), the beam will lack photons of a sufficiently high energy, and be incapable of sufficient penetration.

Beam quality

The braking radiation photons that form most of an X-ray beam's energy, cover a range of values, due to the various distances between the passing filament electrons and the target atoms' nuclei. This mixture of photon energies makes the beam **heterogeneous**; it forms a **continuous spectrum**. Production of maximum energy photons is a rare event: they are only minor contributors to the beam's overall energy (Figure 2.7). So, while the X-ray tube kilovoltage is a very significant factor, it doesn't fully indicate the beam's penetrating potential. A more reliable guide is obtained by considering the full profile of a beam's photon energies. When the maximum photon energy is well supported by medium-to-high photon energies, the beam's penetrating potential is greater than when the other photon energies in the beam have lower values. A beam's photon energy distribution determines what is known as its **quality**.

Graphical display of bremsstrahlung's continuous spectrum shows both positive and negative slopes: across the range of photon energies, from minimum to maximum, relative intensities first increase, then decrease. Between these two features, lies a point of equilibrium, associated with maximum relative intensity. This indicates the beam's **modal** photon energy – and its quality.

In addition to the tube kilovoltage, another important influence on beam quality must be mentioned: primary beam **filtration**

Two

electrons are accelerated across the tube, from cathode to anode, through an applied potential difference, measured in kilovolts. So, if an X-ray tube is operated at 75 kV, electrons crossing the tube will reach the target with 75 keV of kinetic energy. If there is 100% conversion of energy, a 75 keV photon of X-ray energy will be produced; in the circumstances, this will be the maximum photon energy.

Note: The concept of a variable 'maximum photon energy' relates only to braking radiation. Characteristic radiation photons have fixed energies, unchangeable by adjustment of the tube kilovoltage – but these too are measured in keV, derived from the electron binding energies of the tube target element(s).

Quality

This term, indirectly expressing the modal photon energy within an X-ray beam, indicates its overall penetrating potential. It takes into account the beam's range of photon energies and their relative intensities. The principal influences on quality are the tube kilovoltage and the beam's filtration. (White light can have a visible 'quality': it may appear 'warm', if there is an increased intensity of long-wavelength colours (e.g. red) or 'cold', if the short-wavelength (blue) end of the spectrum is more conspicuous.)

It is important not to confuse this scientific meaning with its everyday usage. X-ray beam quality may be *high* or *low*; it is inappropriate to describe it as either 'good' or 'poor'.

In clinical practice, diagnostic X-ray beam quality is informally indicated simply by quoting the tube kilovoltage. More accurately, it is measured at a given kilovoltage, according to the thickness in millimetres of sheet metal (usually aluminium) which reduces the intensity of the beam to 50% of its original value: termed the 'half-value layer'.

Filtration

An X-ray beam is heterogeneous. While its higher photon energies penetrate the object and pass through to the image receptor with sufficient intensity to form an image, its lower values, with less penetrating potential, may be incapable of reaching the image

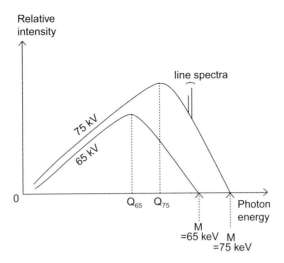

Figure 2.7 The effect on X-ray production of *a kilovoltage increase*. The increase from 65 kV to 75 kV adds energy to the beam. The maximum bremsstrahlung photon energy, M (in kiloelectron volts, numerically equal to the tube kilovoltage), increases from 65 keV to 75 keV, raising the modal value Q (the beam's quality). The increased energy, with the photons' extra penetration, raises beam intensity ($I \propto kV^2$). There is one further change: the production of k characteristic radiation – represented by two line spectra. The k-shell binding energy of tungsten is approximately 69.5 keV. So, filament electrons accelerated across the tube at 65 kV, *having 65 keV kinetic energy*, cannot remove k-shell electrons from atoms in the tube target. But at 75 kV, k-shell characteristic radiation *is* produced; the line spectra demonstrate the beam's increased intensity at two specific energy values, due to photons produced by l → k and m → k transitions.

(Figure 2.8). Unlike tube kilovoltage, filtration normally cannot be changed; it must satisfy a minimum value specified by law, and its purpose concerns the patient's safety rather than beam penetration. So, in practice, beam quality is controlled by the tube kilovoltage alone. When kV is raised, higher X-ray photon energies are added to the beam, increasing its quality. Conversely, when a lower kV value is selected, the upper limit of photon energies is reduced, causing a drop in the modal value: i.e. beam quality decreases.

Beam intensity

In considering beam quality, the relative intensities of the various photon energies across the X-ray spectrum have been mentioned. But their combined effect, i.e. the intensity of the whole beam, is equally important. It is defined as the *rate of flow of X-ray energy through unit measuring area set at right angles to the path of the beam.*

Two

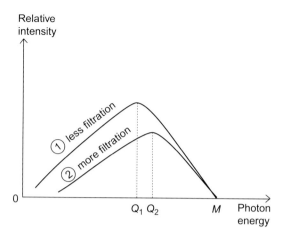

Figure 2.8 The effect on X-ray production of *an increase in beam filtration*. Extra filtration increases the selective elimination of low-energy photons from the beam, raising the modal value, Q (the beam's quality). The maximum photon energy, dependent on the tube kilovoltage, is *unchanged*. Because filtration removes energy, there is an intensity reduction, affecting the beam's lower photon energies more than the higher (consistent with its radiation protection purpose). For simplicity, only bremsstrahlung has been considered, but the intensity of characteristic radiation is similarly reduced.

Although the atomic number of the tube target material and the amount of filtration both affect an X-ray beam's intensity, they are principally concerned, respectively, with X-ray production *efficiency* and radiation *safety*, and will be discussed later, under these headings.

The two controllable influences on the intensity of the X-ray beam emitted from the tube are the tube current (mA) and kilovoltage. Beam intensity at a point remote from the tube – e.g. at the plane where an image is formed, within the image receptor – depends on its distance from the X-ray tube target.

Tube current

Tube current variation (by selection) is the preferred method of controlling X-ray beam intensity because this relationship is simple and direct (Figure 2.9). Beam intensity is determined by the rate at which X-ray energy is emitted from the tube. This output is *directly proportional* to the rate at which electrons bring kinetic energy to the target (its input). The rate at which electrons reach the target is measured as the tube current.

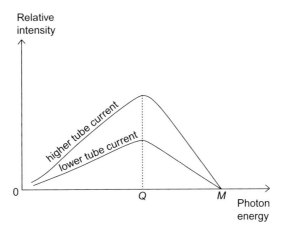

Figure 2.9 The effect on X-ray production of a *reduction in the tube current (mA)*. X-ray tube current (mA) is a measure of the rate of flow of electrons across the tube – and is so also the rate of arrival of electrons, bombarding the tube's target. This has a direct effect on the rate of X-ray production – and the beam's intensity ($I \propto$ mA). *There are no changes to the beam's maximum photon energy or its quality.* (For simplicity again, only bremsstrahlung is considered but mA reduction similarly reduces the intensity of characteristic radiation.)

Tube kilovoltage

Tube kV selection is normally concerned with controlling the beam's quality but it also has an automatic influence on beam intensity. Again, the relationship has a simple basis: the tube's output rate is proportional to its energy input rate. While tube current (mA) indicates the rate at which electrons reach the tube target, the kilovoltage determines the amount of *energy per electron*. So the tube's energy output rate – the beam intensity – depends on kV as well as mA: it is *directly proportional to the squared value* of the kilovoltage.

Distance

An X-ray beam's intensity varies according to where measurement is made, relative to the X-ray tube. As a measuring point is moved further away from the tube's focal spot, intensity reduces in proportion to the *squared value* of the distance: it obeys an **inverse square law** (Figure 2.10).

For special purposes, dose measurements and calculations can usefully be made at points within the patient's body. But the most significant and practical place at which to measure intensity – e.g. for the purpose of automatically timing an exposure – is at or adjacent to the image receptor.

Two

receptor. Exposure to these can bring no benefit to the patient: they only contribute to the radiation dose and increase the patient's 'risk'.

This situation is addressed by the use of a primary beam filter: a thin sheet of aluminium (atomic number 13) across the tube window, easily penetrated by most of the high-energy photons but sufficiently opaque to absorb a significant proportion of low-energy photons, preventing them from reaching the patient. Primary X-ray beam filtration is required by law.

Intensity

This X-ray beam parameter is defined as the rate of flow of energy through unit measuring area, set at 90° to the direction of the approaching beam. This is similar to a definition of light or sound intensity – though in these cases, reference would be made to the *brightness* of the light or the *loudness* of the sound.

Inverse square law

As an X-ray measuring device is moved further away from the source, the intensity of the beam is found to reduce. This is similar to a sound's decreasing loudness or a light's decreasing brightness; it occurs because of the widening spread of the energy. The relationship between X-ray intensity and distance requires accurate investigation – achievable because X-ray beam intensity is governed by an inverse square law. Three conditions apply:

(1) The radiation should be emitted from a *point source*. This is not strictly true (because it is impossible) but an X-ray tube's focal spot is so small in comparison to most practical measuring distances, that this discrepancy is overlooked.

(2) The source must be *isotropic*. This means that its emissions must be equal in all directions. This is actually true – X-ray photons are emitted from the tube target, in all directions – though, in practice, it may fail to be recognised because photons directed into the mass of the anode are wasted by absorption; only photons emerging from the target face have any practical use. Even then, only a small fraction of the photons – those travelling towards the tube window – are useable. (A common example of a *non-isotropic* source is a

car headlight: the bulb is backed by a reflector that directs all its emissions forwards, as an intensified beam.)

(3) There should be *no attenuation*, while the beam passes between its source and the measuring point. To meet this condition strictly, a vacuum would be required. In practice, attenuation in air is minimal and can be disregarded.

If the radiation source is considered to lie at the centre of a series of imaginary spheres, the emitted energy diverging from its source, encounters the walls of the spheres, in turn, each larger that the previous one. So, as the radial distance increases, the emitted energy is spread more sparsely over the spheres' walls. In other words, intensity reduces.

The reduction per unit area (the way in which intensity is defined) is controlled by the relationship between the surface area of a sphere (A) and its radius (r): $A = 4/3\pi r^2$. Discounting the constants in this equation, the surface area of a sphere increases in direct proportion to the squared value of its radius. So, the intensity of the emitted radiation decreases inversely with the squared value of the distance between its source and the measuring point.

What is the practical relevance of the Inverse Square law (ISL)?

The ISL explains the link between (i) focus–image distance, and (ii) the mAs value required to form a radiographic image – i.e. the product of tube current (mA) and exposure time (s) at a given kV. When standardised distances are used, consideration of the ISL may arguably be of minor importance. But when a focus–image distance has to be changed, unless an automatic exposure device is used, the mAs factor has to be recalculated, in relation to the squared value of the focus–image distance. An easy-to-remember example is that if the focus–image distance is changed by a factor of 2, the mAs has to be changed by a factor of 2^2 – i.e. by 4 – *not* by 2.

When the focus–image distance is changed, shouldn't the kV be changed, too?

Normally, the kV should only be changed when more or less penetration is required. This requirement is unaffected by altering the length of the X-ray beam's path through air, between the tube and the object. It should be remembered, also, that a change in kV has an effect on image contrast.

Commentary

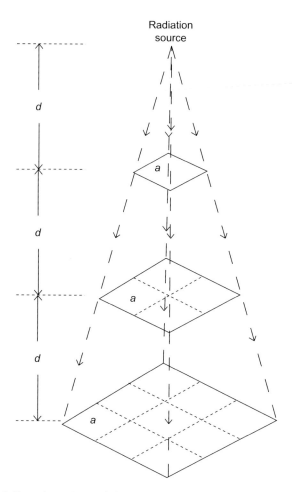

Figure 2.10 X-ray intensity and the inverse square law. As distance increases, between radiation source and measuring plane (the beam's cross-section), the diverging photon beam is spread across an increasingly large area. The growth of this area is directly proportional to the squared value of the distance: *a* at *d*, 4*a* at 2*d*, and 9*a* at 3*d*. So, defined as *the rate of flow through unit area*, intensity is inversely proportional to the squared value of the distance from the source.

Focal spot size

X-rays are produced within an area on the anode bombarded by the electron stream from the filament. This cannot be infinitely small – i.e. a 'point source' – because although the focusing cup's action is precise, it cannot direct all the electrons from the filament to an infinitely small point. So the X-ray source has an identifiable size, which is why all images, in theory, have a measure of geometric unsharpness.

Most diagnostic X-ray tubes are '**dual focus**': the X-ray beam can be produced from either of two sources. These are normally of different sizes: the larger is termed 'broad', the smaller 'fine'. To create these two focal spots, the cathode has two filaments, each within its separate focusing cup. Focal spot size is selected by connecting a heating voltage to one filament or the other. Unless it is linked automatically to another function, focal spot selection appears as a feature on the generator's control panel. The choice between 'fine' or 'broad' focus has a direct effect on the penumbra formed within the X-ray beam when it penetrates an object. It also influences the maximum safe X-ray output rate, in response to the problem of heat production. Heat production within a smaller volume raises its temperature more quickly than if the volume is larger. So, when fine focus is in use, stricter limits have to be imposed on the rate of X-ray production than when broad focus is used.

Smaller focal spot sizes are appropriate for limiting geometric unsharpness in images of securely immobilised, easily penetrated objects. Otherwise, particularly if there is a likelihood of movement during the exposure, a larger focal spot will be selected, enabling beam intensity to be higher, and exposure time to be shorter.

Cross-sectional area

Adjustment of the X-ray beam's cross-sectional area, by widening or narrowing the aperture through which it emerges, is termed **collimation** (Figure 2.11). The X-ray **field**'s size and shape are varied according to the object: a large anatomical area, such as the abdomen, requires a more extensive field than a hand or elbow. The field must always lie entirely within the input borders of the image receptor: any excess represents negligence, imposing extra risk on the patient, with no opportunity for gaining benefit in return. If possible, field size is reduced until it covers the required anatomical parts only, and its shape may be modified to give the patient further protection and limit formation of **scatter**.

X-ray equipment allows these five beam parameters and its other functions to be controlled accurately, efficiently and safely. X-ray production and control are now reviewed from these three perspectives.

Accuracy of X-ray production and control

Introduction

Accuracy of X-ray production is important, especially when radiographic (single, stationary) images are being exposed because, in a

The effect of kilovoltage on X-ray beam intensity

Two factors underlie this relationship, summarised by the equation $I \propto (kV)^2$.

(1) The kilovoltage determines the kinetic energy of the electron stream from the filament that bombards the tube target – and so also the energy of the X-ray photons – i.e. the higher the kV, the higher the X-ray production rate.

(2) From their origins in the tube's target, the photons' efficiency in penetrating the filtration and leaving the tube, to form part of the beam, depends on their energy – i.e. the higher the kV, the higher the output rate.

Can the effect of kV change on beam intensity be useful?

Yes. Although a kV increase tends to reduce image contrast, the accompanying increase in beam intensity can be useful if there is a particular need to reduce exposure time – i.e. when the reduction of movement unsharpness diagnostically outweighs a loss of contrast. An example would be a situation when respiratory movement is difficult to control. The change is easiest to achieve when an automatic exposure device is used. Otherwise, the exposure time reduction has to be calculated or based on previous experience. (An old radiographic 'rule of thumb' suggests a halving of the mAs value, to accompany an increase by 10 kV.)

Dual focus

A dual focus X-ray tube has two specified focal spot sizes, usually different: for example, 1.2 millimetres square and 0.6 millimetres square, commonly referred to as the tube's 'broad' and 'fine' foci. The dual-focus facility is due to having two filaments within the cathode. They lie within separate focusing cups and are fed by separate voltages, based on size and age (state of wear). This arrangement effectively offers the user a choice of two X-ray tubes: one for when reduction of X-ray penumbra is critical for ensuring optimum image quality; the other for when a high X-ray intensity is more important.

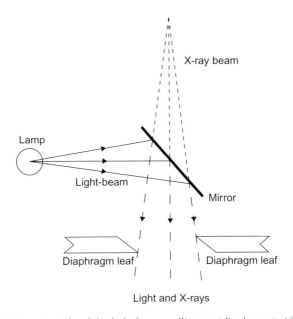

X-ray beam

Lamp

Light-beam

Mirror

Diaphragm leaf

Diaphragm leaf

Light and X-rays

Figure 2.11 The principle of the light-beam collimator (diaphragm). After passing through the radiolucent mirror set at 45° to the central ray, the X-ray beam is joined by a reflected, visible light beam. Both are then cropped and shaped by a system of radiopaque leaves, to give a visible indication *before the exposure*, of the X-ray field's centring, shape and size. The accuracy of this arrangement is critical. Any disturbance of the mirror's angulation creates a collimation error, so its early detection by a regular QA check, is crucial to both the benefits and risks involved in the patient's examination.

sense, these procedures are 'blind'. An image receptor is exposed with skill and care but it isn't until the image has been processed and viewed that the accuracy of the exposure – and the image's diagnostic value – can be confirmed. Uncertainty is minimised if care has been taken to ensure that the X-ray equipment is functioning accurately. Responsibility for accuracy is shared: manufacturers contribute their equipment's reliability; operators must use it correctly and carefully, observing a rigorous **Quality Assurance** scheme. Some relevant points are now considered, starting with the energy input.

Mains voltage compensation

Most X-ray generators receive their energy from the mains voltage supply (Figure 2.12). The reliability of this input tends to be taken for granted but, in practice, occasional variations occur. Mains

Two

Note: The two filaments do not act as 'one and a spare'. Focal spot size has no effect on the X-ray field size: this is determined by collimation and distance from the tube.

Isn't fine focus better than broad focus?

The answer depends on the circumstances. Focus selection should follow anticipation of the likeliest cause of unsharpness.

■ If the object is easily penetrated and easily immobilised, geometric unsharpness may be prominent – and it can be reduced by use of the fine focus.

■ If immobilisation is going to be a potential problem, a high X-ray intensity will allow the exposure time to be minimised. A broad focus (which can safely accept higher rates of heat production) allows higher tube current values to be used, and exposure times to be shortened.

Collimation

This term describes the adjustment, usually in the sense of reduction, of an X-ray beam's cross-sectional area. The beam passing through the X-ray tube's window requires collimation, essentially to lie within the boundaries of the image receptor; then further, to cover just the anatomical area being examined. Collimation is normally performed by use of a light-beam collimator (or 'diaphragm') but, in specialised cases, a fixed diaphragm or a cylindrical cone may be preferred.

Field

This is the area exposed to X-rays, normally measured or specified at an identified distance from the X-ray tube.

Light beam collimator (diaphragm)

This standard device, fitted to most diagnostic X-ray tubes, offers:

■ a wide variety of X-ray fields, to suit all circumstances – e.g. size of anatomical area, image receptor size and shape, focus–image distance variation;

- indication, by illumination, of the X-ray field while its size is being adjusted before an exposure is made;
- accurate confirmation of where the X-ray beam is centred.

An electric lamp, positioned away from the X-ray beam, has its light reflected by a mirror exactly along the X-ray beam's path, through a set of adjustable collimating shutters. These are usually symmetrical, opposing metal plates, producing a rectangular field, to match the shape of the image receptor. See Figure 2.11.

Alternatively, the leaves may be arranged to create a circular iris, forming a better match for the shape of some anatomical structures.

Scatter

This is secondary X-radiation, emanating from an irradiated object, not from the X-ray tube. Scatter has two main characteristics: its direction is random (unlike the predictable, straight-from-the-tube-target, primary beam) and its photon energies tend to be lower than the primary photons.

Quality assurance

In its widest context, quality assurance concerns the formulation of a programme of production principles, standards and methods, so rigorous that imperfections are most unlikely (ideally, never) to be found in the 'products'. In diagnostic radiography, the 'product' is naturally interpreted as the diagnostic image, so a diagnostic radiography QA programme will aim to:

- conduct a patient's X-ray investigation so that it yields the maximum amount of diagnostic information, while
- exposing patients to the minimum amount of X-ray energy ('as low as reasonably practicable').

The achievement of both these aims depends on accurate equipment function, because the difficulty of recognising radiation abnormalities (owing to its invisibility, etc.) and the brevity of exposure times, make reactive correction impossible.

Note: Quality assurance is essentially preventative, not reactive.

Commentary

Nominal values

These are stated 'correct' or ideal values. The term tends to be used under circumstances where there is a possibility that the ideal might not necessarily be achieved. For example, mains voltage is quoted as a nominal value because varying consumer demands during the course of the day can, within narrow limits, temporarily reduce its value or allow it to drift higher.

Fluctuations

This term describes the variations in mains voltage that occur when actual values occasionally rise above or fall below the nominal value.

Transformer

This is an electrical device used to change the value of an alternating voltage: either to increase it (a 'step-up' transformer) or reduce it (a 'step-down' transformer).

A transformer is normally composed of two lengths of insulated wire, both wound around its central, soft iron core. These two windings are electrically separate from each other, and each operates at a different voltage. The input voltage (the value to be changed) is applied across the transformer's primary winding. The required output voltage is electromagnetically induced across the secondary winding. The ratio between input and output voltages is established by the relative number of turns of the primary and secondary windings, around the iron core – termed the *turns ratio*.

The X-ray generator's high-voltage transformer steps-up its input to the required kilovoltage. X-ray tube filaments operate from relatively low voltages, supplied by step-down, tube filament transformers. (In recent years, small, step-down transformers have become widely familiar through their use in mobile phone battery chargers.)

Ohm's law

The 19th-century German physicist, Georg Ohm, performed and published experimental work to confirm the relationship between a voltage (potential difference) applied across a metallic conductor and the resultant current that flows through it.

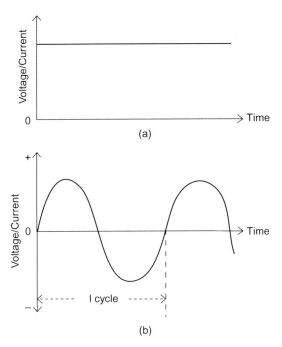

Figure 2.12 Types of voltage and current. (a) A direct voltage, such as produced by a battery, has a fixed (positive/negative) polarity and a constant magnitude. When applied across a conductor, it produces a direct current, flowing in a single direction, with a constant magnitude. (Its value depends on the conductor's resistance.) (b) An alternating voltage, such as that obtained from a mains supply, has a constantly changing magnitude, between zero and the peak value, and a periodically reversing polarity. When applied across a simple conductor, it produces an alternating current, which has a constantly changing magnitude (normally in phase with the applied voltage) and a periodically reversing direction.

voltages are normally quoted as **nominal values**. When circumstances are ideal, the value of the supplied voltage actually matches this figure. At other times, it may be slightly under or above the nominal value. These spontaneous variations are termed **fluctuations**. They seldom affect the operation of household electrical appliances but (in the absence of compensation) their influence on X-ray equipment output could be serious, affecting beam quality and intensity, and reducing image contrast.

X-ray generators contain a voltage-sensitive device that continuously monitors the input voltage. Most generators respond automatically to feedback from this device, ensuring that generator output remains constant, whatever the actual value of the mains supply. But some older or more basic generators have manually-operated mains voltage compensators. These depend on (i) the operator's alert observation of a mains voltage indicator on the

The current (the consequence) is directly proportional to the voltage (the cause), provided that the physical condition of the conductor remains constant. The proportional current rise that accompanies an increased potential difference is explained by the fact that a metallic conductor – a copper wire, for example – contains an immense reserve of relatively free electrons, ready to respond (by joining the flow) when the voltage is increased.

Saturation

Copper wire contains a virtually unlimited supply of electrons, available to flow as a current, when a voltage is connected across the wire, as part of an electrical circuit. In contrast to this, when operating as a component in its high-voltage circuit, an X-ray tube's only source is its heated filament, which emits electrons at a rate controlled by its temperature. During an exposure, the kilovoltage applied across an X-ray tube is so high in proportion to the rate at which the filament is emitting electrons, that all are accelerated across to the anode at this same rate. Even if the kV is increased, the filament will not emit electrons at a higher rate than its temperature allows; Ohm's law does not apply. The important practical effect of saturation is that the current (mA) across the X-ray tube is independent of the applied tube kilovoltage.

(Other instances of saturation are found elsewhere in scientific practice. For example, when all the domains within a magnetic specimen have been aligned to the imposed lines of force, its magnetic strength cannot be increased: it is saturated.)

Automatic exposure control

If the object being X-rayed is relatively opaque (large, dense), significant X-ray attenuation occurs. Consequently, the intensity of the emergent X-ray beam is relatively low. An automatic exposure device (AED) measures this low intensity and proportionately delays the end of the exposure until sufficient X-ray energy has reached the image receptor, to form a latent image.

Alternatively, if the object is relatively radiolucent (thin, easily penetrated) the emergent X-ray beam is more intense. This higher intensity activates the AED to bring the exposure to an early conclusion – again producing a correctly exposed image.

control panel and then (ii) simple adjustment of a control, to make compensations when required.

Accuracy and independence of selected kilovoltage

The tube kilovoltage may be four or five hundred times higher than the mains voltage. The required multiplication is produced by the generator's **high-voltage transformer**, which 'steps up' the voltages supplied to it (selected at the control panel) into kilovoltages for connection across the X-ray tube. When the transformer operates (for the duration of the exposure only) significant energy losses occur within the generator that would seriously disturb the accuracy of the kV, if it were not for the compensation circuit. This calculates the side-effects in advance (which occur in proportion to the selected mA) and adjusts the voltage supplied to the high-voltage transformer, so that when the exposure is made, the kV is exactly as selected, whether the mA is high or low. This independence is essential to the accuracy of the X-ray beam's quality and intensity.

Accuracy and independence of tube current

Unlike much electrical equipment, X-ray tubes don't operate according to **Ohm's law**: tube current is *not* directly proportional to tube kilovoltage (Figure 2.13). It is true that a kilovoltage is necessary for producing the tube current: without a potential difference between anode and cathode, no current would flow. But in practice, tube current is solely controlled by the rate at which free electrons are made available from the heated filament; the mA selector on the generator's control panel actually controls the filament's temperature.

Tube current selection is supported by complex circuitry. This operates so accurately that the filament's rate of electron emission *exactly* matches the selected current. It includes a compensator, which ensures that the X-ray tube operates under **saturation** conditions: *mA is independent of kV*. These circumstances are essential for precise control of X-ray beam intensity, and for preventing thermal damage to the tube's anode.

Radiographic exposure timing

For radiographic purposes (as opposed to fluoroscopy – where there are different requirements) every X-ray generator has an

Two

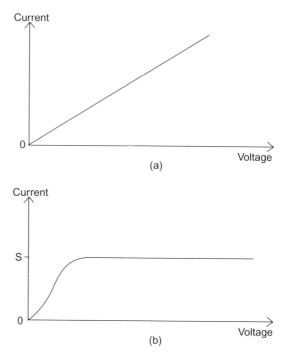

Figure 2.13 Ohm's law and saturation. (a) Ohm's law states that the application of a voltage across a simple conductor, such as a copper wire, in a constant physical state, produces a proportional current through it. The proportionality (determined by the conductor's resistance) holds true across a potentially large range of voltages, from zero upwards, until there is a change in the conductor's physical conditions – e.g. its temperature. (b) The application of a voltage across an appliance, such as an X-ray tube, where conduction is reliant on the controlled availability of electrons, e.g. by thermionic emission from a filament, also produces a current. But in this case, a rise in the voltage can increase the current only until it reaches the rate at which electrons are being made available. At this point, S, the current is said to become *saturated*; it cannot increase further, however high the voltage. Only a rise in the rate of electron supply, e.g. due to a higher filament temperature, will enable the current to increase. The X-ray generator control circuit that ensures X-ray tube current is independent of the selected kilovoltage, is based on this principle.

exposure timer. Manual operation enables the operator to select 0.001 second or 0.3 second or whatever is considered appropriate. Pressing the 'exposure' button simultaneously:

(a) applies the selected kilovoltage across the X-ray tube;
(b) starts the exposure timer.

The function of the timer is to switch off the X-ray exposure after the selected period of time.

Even though exposure timers are accurate and reliable, manual selection of exposure times, whether based on the operator's experience or a standardised guide, is becoming less common. It tends to be limited to X-ray examinations of the limbs, and a few other instances when correct estimation of exposure requirements is fairly easy – where variations from 'normal' are minor and familiar.

Compared with these, examinations of the thorax and abdomen may pose difficulties: accurate pre-selection of exposure times can be frustrated by unpredictable, abnormal radiopacities or radio-lucencies. If errors produce incorrectly exposed images, the potential consequences include:

▓ reduced diagnostic information, weakening the *benefit* available in return for the *risk*; and
▓ in some instances, a need to repeat the exposure – which seriously disrupts the *benefit versus risk* relationship, by effectively doubling the *risk*.

Repeat exposures also unnecessarily waste time and materials, and can cause the patient further inconvenience and emotional stress. All these inefficiencies can be prevented by the use of an **automatic exposure device** (AED – see Figure 2.14). As an exposure proceeds, the AED monitors the emergent X-ray beam, at a plane just before the beam reaches the image receptor. The AED's action is to terminate the exposure when a sufficient quantity of radiation, programmed beforehand, has been absorbed by the image receptor. This quantity is based on an expectation that it will form an image of the required density or brightness (depending on the type of image receptor and the viewing mode).

Monitoring is normally achieved by measuring the ionisation that occurs while the emergent beam passes through a volume of air, held within a sealed radiolucent chamber.

X-ray production efficiency

Introduction

It is hard to claim, by normal standards, that an X-ray tube is 'efficient'. If efficiency is measured by expressing *useful* energy output as a percentage of energy input, a tube suffers from three serious weaknesses:

Two

Automatic timers are familiar devices when built into photographic cameras. Their action is to monitor light intensity (from the intended scene or subject) before an exposure is made and feed this information back to the camera's aperture or shutter. In comparison, the monitoring of X-ray intensity is more complicated: it cannot be undertaken until an exposure starts, and several precautions are necessary, to ensure reliable operation.

These include:

■ calibrating the device to the speed of the image receptor (the AED is only capable of measuring X-ray energy, not its visible consequences);

■ relating the monitoring area correctly to the patient's body – this usually involves both positioning the patient and selection of an appropriately sited monitoring chamber;

■ pre-selecting an ideal image density, which effectively programmes the device to end the exposure when a given quantity of X-ray energy has reached the image receptor; and

■ ensuring no accidentally misleading conditions or equipment settings can produce a falsely short or over-prolonged exposure time.

During X-ray production, how many photons are produced?

It depends on the circumstances: kilovoltage, efficiency of the target, type of generator, etc. Here are just a few numbers:

■ If the X-ray tube current is 500 mA, 0.5 coulombs of electric charge pass across the tube per second.

■ One coulomb of negative charge equates to approximately 6×10^{18} electrons.

■ When the tube current is 500 mA, three million million million electrons cross the tube per second.

■ Even if only 5% of these have their kinetic energy converted into X-rays, this involves one hundred and fifty thousand million million electrons every second.

Atomic number

The atomic number of an element is the number of protons within the nucleus of each of its atoms. In a neutral atom, the atomic number equally indicates the number of orbiting electrons.

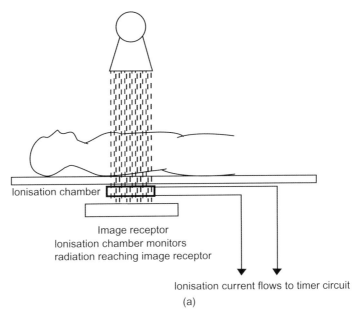

Ionisation chamber

Image receptor
Ionisation chamber monitors
radiation reaching image receptor

Ionisation current flows to timer circuit

(a)

Two

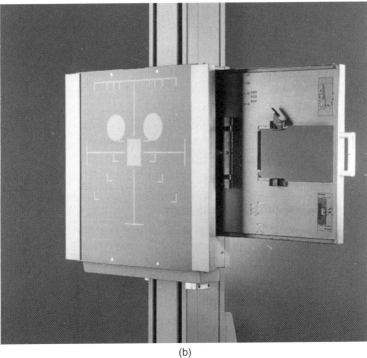

(b)

Figure 2.14 An automatic exposure device. (a) Detector chambers are located between the patient and the image receptor. (b) Their shape and position within the field can be indicated on the front panel of a table or vertical bucky (as shown) or projected through a pattern imprinted on the light beam collimator's window (photograph by courtesy of Philips Medical Systems).

(1) X-ray photons are emitted from the tube target in all direc-tions, so only a fraction of them travel usefully towards and through the tube window. X-rays cannot be focused or re-directed, so this situation has to be accepted. The potential radiation hazard presented by X-rays travelling in other direc-tions (except towards the window) is prevented by a lining of sheet lead, within the tube housing.

(2) Inherent in bremsstrahlung production is the fact that many of the X-ray photons emerging from tube's target have too little energy to penetrate the object and contribute to image formation. Again, in addition to poor efficiency, this presents a radiation hazard: low-energy photons that are absorbed superficially, increase the patient's risk but cannot add to the benefit. This problem is principally reduced by the use of primary beam filtration.

(3) Of the electron stream's kinetic energy reaching the tube target, typically less than 5% is converted into X-ray energy. The remainder is converted into heat. Again, this shortcoming is inherent: it cannot be resolved. However, X-ray tubes and generators incorporate features that, within limits, restrict this inefficiency. Some of these will now be described.

Energy conversion efficiency

When a filament electron interacts with a target atom to produce an X-ray photon, three main factors determine an individual photon's energy.

(1) The electron's path in relation to either:
  – the atom's nucleus – to produce a photon of braking radiation, or
  – the atom's orbiting electrons – to produce characteristic radiation.

(2) The electron's kinetic energy – the initial energy available for conversion.

(3) The target element's **atomic number** – which controls both the strength of the atom's nuclear field and its electron (shell) binding energy values.

Control of the filament electron stream

The cathode's focusing cup shapes the stream of electrons emitted from the filament, so that they bombard only a specified area on the surface of the anode, the target. If the tube's 'broad focus' has been selected, the target's area is very small; if 'fine' focus is in use, it is even smaller. But greater accuracy, as previously mentioned, is impossible. So, it is a matter of chance whether an electron will (a) pass close enough to an atomic nucleus to experience a sudden force, or (b) hit an orbiting electron and remove it from its shell, or (c) produce nothing except a contribution to anode heating. The likelihood of this last option far outweighs that of the first two.

The filament electrons' kinetic energy

Electrons crossing the X-ray tube derive their kinetic energy from the kilovoltage applied across the tube: the higher the kV, the faster the electrons travel towards the tube's target. For a given value of kV, efficiency is at its highest if the X-ray generator supplies the tube with a direct, 'constant potential' kilovoltage, so that all electrons reach the target with the same kinetic energy – i.e. they are equally able to produce X-ray photons.

An X-ray generator receives an input of a relatively low, **alternating** voltage. This is taken through three principal steps: voltage transformation, kilovoltage rectification, and increase of kilovoltage frequency.

(a) Voltage transformation

The mains voltage supplied to an X-ray generator is much too low to be successfully applied across the X-ray tube, between anode and cathode. The generator's high-voltage transformer produces the required increase, by a factor in the range 400 to 500 (Figure 2.15).

(b) Kilovoltage rectification

Like its input, the output from a transformer is an alternating voltage. For many purposes, an alternating output is acceptable but these do *not* include supplying an X-ray tube with its kilovoltage. Application of an alternating kV across the X-ray tube would give its electrodes a constantly changing polarity. Instead of always being at positive potential to attract filament electrons, the anode would be negative for half of the exposure time, and a similar inefficiency would affect the cathode.

Alternating voltage

This is a voltage that has a constantly changing magnitude and a periodically reversing polarity.

Rectification circuit

Normally, when an alternating voltage is applied across a conductor, an alternating current is produced: electrons travel in one direction (negative to positive) but then in response to the reversed polarity, travel in the opposite direction (*still* negative to positive). A rectifier is a device that permits electrons to flow through it in one direction only, even when an alternating voltage is applied across it.

An X-ray generator's high-voltage rectification circuit contains rectifiers connected together so that by either allowing or blocking electron flow, in turn, they change an applied alternating voltage into a pulsating output voltage with a fixed polarity.

Out of phase/In phase

Properties that change their values throughout a cycle, such as alternating voltages and currents, are described as being 'in phase' when they reach zero and their peak values simultaneously. When properties lack this harmony, they are described as being 'out of phase'.

Frequency

This indicates the rate at which a given property or value goes through a regular cycle of change. When applied to an alternating voltage or an electromagnetic radiation, the term 'frequency' effectively means 'cycles per second'.

The SI unit of frequency is the hertz (symbol, Hz).

Overload prevention

An X-ray tube can only tolerate heat production up to a given, safe limit, imposed by its thermal capacity and the rate at which cooling

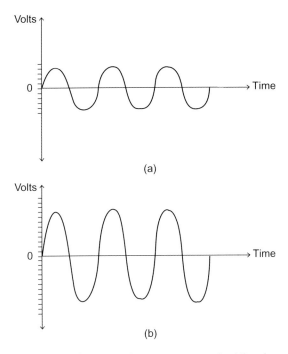

Figure 2.15 Conversion of mains voltage into X-ray tube kilovoltage – 1: transformation. Transformation of an alternating voltage from a lower value (a) to a higher (b) raises its (peak) magnitude, according to the transformer's *turns ratio*. A transformer's secondary (output) voltage is a fixed multiple of the primary (input) voltage.

To operate efficiently, an X-ray tube must be fed with a kilovoltage of fixed polarity, so that its anode is consistently positive and its cathode negative (Figure 2.16). This requirement is met by the use of a **rectification circuit**, located between the high-voltage transformer and the X-ray tube.

(c) Increase of kilovoltage frequency

Even when rectified, a pulsating kilovoltage, varying between zero and the peak value, falls short of being ideal. X-ray photons capable of forming an image will not normally be produced until the kV across the tube, rising from zero, reaches about 45 kV; and production will cease when it falls below this value again, as it approaches zero. So, although rectification ensures consistent kV polarity, it doesn't prevent X-ray production from being intermittent; between X-ray pulses, the electrons' kinetic energy is only (and unprofitably) converted into heat.

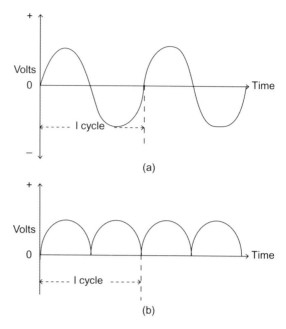

Figure 2.16 Conversion of mains voltage into X-ray tube kilovoltage – 2: rectification. Rectifiers, devices designed to allow current to flow through them in one specific direction only, are used to convert an alternating voltage (a) into a supply that has a constant polarity. The simplest arrangement just excludes alternate 'inverse' half-cycles, but a more efficient system reverses these half-cycles, so that – with this single-phase supply – there are two 'forward' voltage pulses per cycle (b). Rectification of the high-voltage transformer's output enables a constant polarity kilovoltage to be applied across the X-ray tube: the anode is always positive, and the cathode negative.

The time intervals between rectified kilovoltage peaks are shortened by two methods: one depends on the type of voltage supply; the other is the result of modification by the generator (Figure 2.17).

Use of a three-phase supply: Mains voltage is distributed from electricity generating stations as three simultaneous, identical supplies, **out of phase** with each other by an interval of a third of a cycle. Houses are normally allocated just a single-phase voltage but larger buildings, including hospitals, receive a three-phase supply. X-ray generators (except for mobile and low-powered units) are fed all three phases. Each phase is transformed and rectified, shortening the time interval between the peaks, eliminating most of the lower values until it becomes a near-constant supply, affected only by a small 'ripple'.

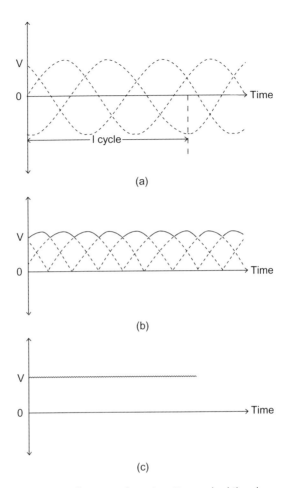

Figure 2.17 Conversion of mains voltage into X-ray tube kilovoltage – 3: increasing the frequency. Rectification of a three-phase voltage supply – three identical voltages separated in time by one-third of a cycle (a) – brings successive pulses closer together than with a single-phase supply, sustaining the voltage within about 10% of its peak value (b). If the original supply frequency (the number of cycles per second) is electronically increased, the rectified form (c) shows virtually no variation in magnitude: the generator's output is a 'constant potential' – effectively a direct kilovoltage, of the selected value. (This is now the standard output from an X-ray generator, making it unnecessary to specify a kilovoltage as a 'peak' value.)

Conversion to high-frequency: Tube kilovoltage ripple is virtually eliminated by increasing its **frequency**. Within the generator, a frequency multiplication circuit raises the supply value – in the UK, 50 hertz – to a value measurable in thousands. This compresses the time dimension of the waveform, effectively converting it into a direct voltage, usually termed a 'constant potential' supply.

The target element's atomic number

An element's atomic number indicates how many protons there are within each of its atoms' nuclei. An element with a relatively high atomic number increases the tube target's efficiency in producing both

■   bremsstrahlung – because its greater nuclear field strength makes more filament electrons undergo sudden changes in direction (Figure 2.18) and

■   characteristic radiation – because the electrons' binding energies are relatively high.

Standard X-ray tube targets are made principally of tungsten. Its atomic number, 74, makes energy conversion to X-rays relatively efficient. But a reasonably high atomic number is not tungsten's only favourable property. It might be imagined that another element – lead, for example, with an atomic number of 82 – could be more efficient as a target material, until the large amount of heat generated during X-ray production is taken into account. Tungsten has the highest melting point of all metallic elements: approximately 3300°C. (Lead melts at 327°C.)

A radiographic interpretation of 'efficiency'

The production of radiographic images (not fluoroscopy) invites a further view of X-ray equipment 'efficiency' – taking into account not only percentage energy conversion but also the *maximum rate* at which conversion (X-ray production) can safely occur. This approach is argued from the basis that in most radiographic situations, a high-intensity X-ray beam is desirable, so that exposure times can be short. A short exposure tends to eliminate movement unsharpness, reinforcing an image's diagnostic value. So, from a radiographic perspective, 'efficient' X-ray equipment is capable of producing a high-intensity X-ray beam. This efficiency is achieved mainly through features of X-ray tube design but also by taking precautions that delay or compensate for a tube's ageing.

High-intensity efficiency *versus* safety

Desirable though it is, a high X-ray output intensity is only available when circumstances allow. The controlling influence is the heat

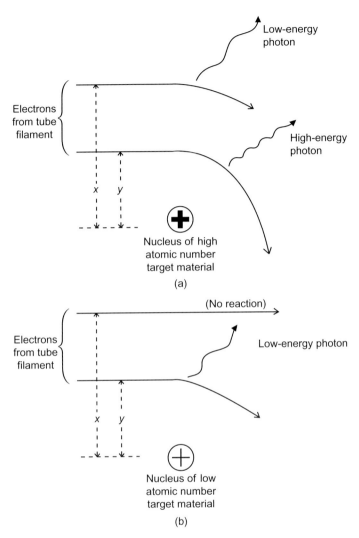

Two

Figure 2.18 Influence on the X-ray beam of *the tube target material's atomic number*. (a) A target material with a relatively high atomic number exerts an attraction on both these filament electrons, potentially converting their kinetic energy into (useful) X-ray energy. (b) A target material with a lower atomic number has a more restricted range of influence. Its conversion of the filament electrons' kinetic energy into X-ray photons is less efficient, producing an X-ray beam that is less intense. In practice, there is little need or opportunity to compare the intensities of X-ray beams produced by different target materials, but comparisons would show that X-ray beam intensity is directly proportional to the target material's atomic number.

Note: Tube target material has no influence on an X-ray beam's quality. This is principally dependent on the kilovoltage and beam filtration.

occurs. If this limit were to be exceeded, thermal damage would occur; the tube would be 'overloaded'.

Overloading is prevented by restrictions on the rate at which electrical energy is supplied to the tube. Maximum safe rates of energy supply are calculated according to the tube's thermal capacity and cooling rates, and the amount of residual heat remaining from previous exposures. Restrictions ensure thermal safety but they also limit the rate at which X-rays can be produced.

Mathematical 'products'

The mathematical meaning of the term *product* is sufficiently different from its everyday usage ('something that is produced') to deserve a brief explanation. In its mathematical sense, a 'product' is simply the outcome of a multiplication.

Milliampere second

This unit is the product of X-ray tube current (measured in milliamperes) and exposure time (in seconds): mA × s = mAs. It indicates a quantity of X-ray energy as an 'exposure factor', at a given kilovoltage.

Its use may be considered strange for the following reasons.

- It is indirect: it is actually a unit of electric *charge*, not X-ray energy. Its validity is argued on the basis that the quantity of electric charge (electrons) reaching the tube target during an exposure determines the quantity of X-radiation produced – i.e. by conversion of their kinetic energy. This is true, for a given energy per electron – i.e. at a stated kV value.
- It is identical to a more widely known unit. Since current is measured as a rate of flow of electric charge (1 milliampere = a flow of 1 millicoulomb per second) multiplication of current by an exposure time, in seconds, yields a quantity of electric charge *in millicoulombs*.

Use of the *milliampere second* in diagnostic radiography can be traced to the convenience of calculating its value simply by multiplying tube current (mA) by exposure time (s). For example, 500 mA × 0.02 s = 10 mAs. Its persistence, in a time when automatic calculation has replaced mental arithmetic, is harder to explain.

created during X-ray productions. It is unfortunate that an increase in the rate of X-ray production is accompanied by a rise in the rate of heat production; heat raises the target's temperature and, despite tungsten's very high melting point, poses a risk of thermal damage. Dangerous situations are avoided by the action of **overload prevention** and exposure control devices, which ensure that all combinations of kV, mA and exposure time are 'safe'. Unfortunately – so far as efficiency is concerned – safety is often achieved only by limiting the X-ray beam's intensity.

At a given kilovoltage, the quantity of X-ray energy required for a radiographic exposure is normally measured using the unit formed when tube current (milliamperes) is multiplied by exposure time (seconds): the **milliampere–second** (symbol: mAs). Safe production of mAs values tends to involve a restricted tube current (mA) and an extended exposure time. The safety of this arrangement is explained by the fact that while the tube target is being heated by the arrival of electrons with their kinetic energy, *it is simultaneously losing heat to its surroundings*. So, as well as being 'a target heating time', an X-ray exposure can be regarded as 'an anode cooling time'. When heated at a reduced rate, using a lower mA, even though the exposure is spread across a longer time, a target will tend not to reach the temperatures that would be produced by a higher heating rate and a shorter cooling time.

It may be argued that even a short extension to the exposure time (to offset an imposed lower mA) could be long enough to allow movement to blur an image. So there is a conflict between efficiency (represented by motion-free images) and safety (represented by an undamaged X-ray tube). Some features of this conflict will emerge during the following account.

Efficiency features of X-ray tube design

Being both the source of the X-ray beam and the area where heat production occurs, an X-ray tube's target:

(a) is positioned in a precise spatial relationship to both the tube's filament and the window;
(b) ideally has a relatively high **thermal capacity**;
(c) is supplied with cooling paths, to draw its heat away.

The fixed anode X-ray tube

The simplest type of X-ray tube has a *fixed* (or *stationary*) anode (Figure 2.19). Though rarely found now in clinical practice, the fixed

Advice to avoid giving scientific symbols a plural 's', is relevant here. There must be no confusion between, for instance, 60 milliamperes (60 mA) and 60 milliampere seconds (60 mAs).

Thermal capacity

This term is defined as the amount of energy (in joules) required to raise the temperature of a given *body* by 1 kelvin (1 Celsius degree).

A body's temperature rise, when heat is introduced, is due to an increase in the rate of vibration of its atoms and molecules. The greater a body's mass, the greater is the amount of heat energy required to take it through a temperature rise of 1 kelvin.

A dental X-ray tube

In circumstances where the search for increased power is the normal trend, the dental X-ray tube used for intra-oral exposures is an anomaly: it has a fixed anode. It is low-powered in the true sense of the word: the rate at which it converts electrical energy into X-ray energy is low – but deliberately so, because the tube is compact, manoeuvrable and relatively inexpensive, and it is used for a specified and very limited range of examinations.

Central ray

X-ray photons are emitted from the face of the target in all (forward) directions. Those that travel through the middle of the tube window and along the central axis of the collimating device form what is termed the 'central ray'. It has no special features except that it is considered to be infinitely thin, non-diverging and so incapable of creating magnification. It is used as an axial reference line when beam angulations are being defined for a given radiographic projection.

Target angle

This is the angle measured between the face of an X-ray tube's target (or the bevelled angle of the anode's focal track) and the axis of the central ray.

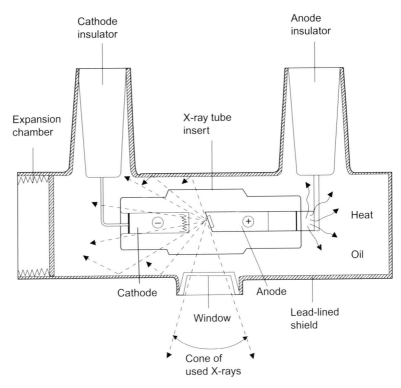

Figure 2.19 A fixed anode X-ray tube (by courtesy of IGE Medical Systems).

anode tube deserves a brief consideration, to introduce the principle of target angulation and to give a background to the advantages of the rotating anode.

Location of the target

The fixed anode's target is a block of tungsten, embedded in the face of a copper cylinder. It is accurately aligned with both the filament within its focusing cup, and the centre of the tube window. The cylinder is held firmly in position by the strength of the glass envelope.

The target's thermal capacity

The face of the copper cylinder, in which the target is embedded, slopes at an angle, oblique to both the cathode and the tube window. Angulation allows free access to the target for the approaching electron stream, and a suitably wide exit path for emerging X-rays. But it also provides a compromise between two conflicting demands.

Two

Thermal conduction

Heat within a solid is characterised by vibration of its atoms and molecules; a rise in temperature indicates an increase in their kinetic energy. Whatever their rate of vibration, provided the material remains solid, the atoms and molecules are unable to change the central points around which they vibrate. Their heat (kinetic) energy affects adjacent molecules, which increase their own rate of vibration. This method of heat transfer is termed conduction. Materials vary according to the efficiency of their thermal conductivity, along a scale from metals, which are efficient thermal conductors, to less efficient materials, through to the least, which may even be regarded as thermal insulators.

Convection

Within a heated gas or a liquid, vibrating particles (atoms and molecules) are free to move, carrying their heat (kinetic) energy to other parts of the body. Vibration loosens the links between particles, allowing expansion of the volume they occupy but without changing their mass; their density (mass per unit volume) decreases and their response to gravity weakens. So, heated particles within gases and liquids tend to rise; the volume they previously occupied is filled by the inward drift of other (colder) particles which, in turn, become hotter and follow the same behaviour. Together, the moving particles form cycles, known as thermal convection currents.

Heat radiation

This is the propagation of heat energy as infra-red electromagnetic radiation – i.e. with energy values lower than in the visible spectrum. As an electromagnetic radiation, it does not need a medium for its propagation: it can cross a vacuum. This fact has practical relevance to X-ray production: the X-ray tube insert is evacuated – so the anode loses its heat, generated as an accompaniment to X-ray production, across the vacuum, to the insert wall.

▪ *Considered as the X-ray source*, there is a strong argument for the target to be *small* – because size limitation restricts penumbra and the image's geometric unsharpness.
▪ *Considered as the area where heat production is concentrated*, there is an equally strong reason why the target should be *large* – because with a greater heat capacity, it is more tolerant of the high rate of heat production that accompanies a high X-ray intensity.

The target area, within which heat and X-rays are produced, is defined by electron focusing. It is actually oblong in shape but, due to foreshortening, if viewed along the axis of the **central X-ray**, it appears to be square and typically only about one-quarter of its actual, oblong size (Figure 2.20). So angulation of the target achieves the required compromise:

▪ its effect on penumbra – and geometric unsharpness – is much less than its true size would produce; *and*
▪ its thermal capacity is retained.

The **target angle**, typically within the range 10° to 15°, controls the ratio between true and effective focal areas – i.e. between the heated area and the area responsible for penumbra. Reduction of the target angle offers a more effective compromise but this advantage cannot be pursued to an extreme, because the sloping face of the target limits the edge of the X-ray beam. (Photons directed behind this boundary are wholly absorbed within the anode.) As the angle approaches zero, the size of the X-ray field becomes limited. If narrowed too much, the field tends to lose its practical usefulness. A tube's effective focal area is better known as the **focus** or **focal spot**, with its size indicated by the dimensions of the square area.

Cooling paths to enable heat to leave the target

The immediate route for heat loss is provided by the target's position within the copper cylinder: it draws heat away from the back and sides of the target, by **conduction**. This operates efficiently because copper has a high **thermal conductivity**, and the cylinder's diameter and length give it a large thermal capacity.

The remote end of the copper cylinder, furthest from the target, protruding into the oil that surrounds the tube insert, is at a relatively low temperature, so heat from the target is conducted

Two

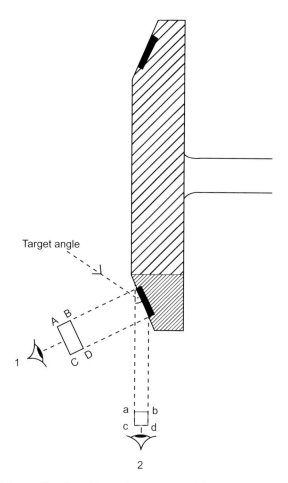

Figure 2.20 Target (focal track) angulation. Viewed face-on (1), the bombarded, X-ray-producing target area has an oblong shape – the 'true focal area' (A-B-C-D), offering the benefit of maximum thermal capacity. When viewed along the central axis of the X-ray beam – the central ray – (2) angulation foreshortens this same area to a square (a-b-c-d), minimising the X-ray penumbra it produces, and the consequent geometric unsharpness. The relationship between these two areas is controlled by the target angle.

towards it. From this point, heat is carried by **convection** to the inner surface of the tube's housing; then, by conduction, through to its outer wall. A smaller loss occurs by **heat radiation** from the target's outer face and the copper cylinder's surface, across the vacuum to the glass envelope from where it is convected via the oil, to the outer parts of the tube. Ultimately, the room's air currents convect heat from the surface of the tube housing.

The rotating anode X-ray tube

The inefficiency of the fixed anode lies in its target's restricted thermal capacity, which severely limits the rate at which X-rays can be produced. The inventor of the rotating anode recognised that:

▦ a distinction can be made between the target's dual functions: the area *where heat is produced* need not be confined to the area *where X-rays are produced*; and

▦ provided that the target remains in a constant position in relation to the focused electron stream and the tube window, X-ray production continues unaffected, even when this bombarded area is in motion.

So, the fixed anode's single, oblong block of tungsten is replaced by the rotating anode's constantly changing oblong area of tungsten – i.e. a small part of its ring-shaped focal track, defined by the limits of electron bombardment. Rotation of the disc carries the recently heated area out of the way of the oncoming electrons, presenting to them a fresh, cooler area, which then itself moves round, making way for another. Although the X-ray source remains the rectangular area directly opposite the tube filament, the ring-shaped focal track heated by filament bombardment may be a hundred or more times larger, with a proportionately increased thermal capacity, and able safely to produce an X-ray beam of much higher intensity.

Two

The focal track's thermal capacity

Factors affecting the thermal capacity of the focal track, the path around the anode's bevelled surface, include: width, length, rotational speed and disc thickness.

Width

The focal track isn't marked by structural boundaries but by electron bombardment. So its width – i.e. the target's length – is effectively determined by the length of the filament, the action of its focusing cup, and the target angle.

Length

Being in the form of a ring, the focal track's 'length' is its mean circumference. This depends on its radial distance from the centre

Specific thermal capacity

The word 'specific' indicates a property of a particular *material*, rather than a (mixed composition) body. This term is defined as the amount of energy required to take 1 kilogram of the material through a temperature rise of 1 kelvin.

Graphite

This is a solid, crystalline form of the element carbon. It has a low atomic number, 6, so it is unsuitable as a target material, but it is ideal for use in the body of the anode disc, with a high specific thermal capacity: $710\,J\,kg^{-1}\,K^{-1}$ (compared with tungsten: $138\,J\,kg^{-1}\,K^{-1}$) and a low density: $2300\,kg\,m^{-3}$ (compared with tungsten: $19\,320\,kg\,m^{-3}$).

Molybdenum

Molybdenum is a metallic element with an atomic number, 42, high enough to enable it to be used as a target material in specialised mammographic X-ray tubes. Its use for this purpose is based on the production of significant, image-forming characteristic radiation to reinforce the bremsstrahlung, even at energies as low as the 20–25 kV employed in mammography. At these kV values, a tungsten target's output would be less efficient.

Molybdenum's more common uses are as the material for the rotating anode stem (it remains strong, even when narrow) and for the body of the anode disc: it has a higher specific thermal capacity than tungsten: $251\,J\,kg^{-1}\,K^{-1}$ (compared with $138\,J\,kg^{-1}\,K^{-1}$) and a lower density: $10\,200\,kg\,m^{-3}$ (compared with $19\,320\,kg\,m^{-3}$).

Temperature gradients

Heat travels 'from a hotter place to a cooler'. A temperature gradient identifies the distance between two such points in a similar way to a physical gradient. A limited comparison may be made to a vehicle free-wheeling down a physical slope: heat travels along a temperature gradient, at a rate proportional to the temperature difference between its ends. A steep temperature gradient will

of the disc, which effectively depends on the disc's diameter. A larger diameter lengthens the focal track – and so increases its thermal capacity – but a larger disc is heavier, and there is more strain on its supporting stem, when rotating. So, large anode discs are not automatic and inevitable features of every X-ray tube. If a tube's workload creates a *regular* need for high thermal capacity, it will be likely to have a relatively large diameter – say, 130 mm. Otherwise a smaller diameter – say, 70 or 80 mm may be in use, on grounds of long-term economy.

Rotational speed

The focal track's 'length' across which the heat of an X-ray exposure is dispersed, depends on the rate at which the disc is rotating. Ideally, electron bombardment should cover all parts of the focal track equally, to take maximum advantage of its thermal capacity. If an exposure time is very short, this condition might not be met: the disc could fail to complete a whole revolution (or whole number of revolutions) before the exposure ends. In this case some of its potential capacity would be unused. To distribute heat more evenly and efficiently, the anode's speed of rotation may be increased – permanently or temporarily, depending on how often this advantage is needed – typically from 3000 up to 10 000 revolutions per minute. But it should be noted that higher speeds are accompanied by increased mechanical wear and extra heat production within the rotation apparatus. Also, the benefits of high-speed rotation diminish as exposure times become longer. So unnecessary use of high speeds should be avoided.

Disc thickness and composition

The disc's thermal capacity may be raised by increasing its thickness. Because this change implies a proportionate increase in its mass and greater mechanical stresses, it is normally accompanied by a change in the composition of the body (the main mass) of the disc. (Its focal track remains the same.) These other materials are chosen for their higher **specific thermal capacities** and relatively lower densities. Both **graphite** and **molybdenum** meet this specification: they can absorb a greater quantity of heat energy per unit temperature rise and (for heat absorption) offer a larger volume per unit mass than tungsten. But both lack tungsten's high atomic number, so they are employed in forming the body of the disc only. On account of both its high melting point and high atomic number, tungsten is retained as the principal focal track material.

Two

make heat travel relatively quickly – but as the two end temperatures become closer, *the gradient reduces* and the rate of heat travel
slows down, until equilibrium is reached and the gradient
disappears.

Electrical resistance

Electrons, forming an electric current, lose energy as they flow
through a conductor, as a result of colliding with the conductor's
atoms. The opposition that an electrical conductor presents, in this
way, is termed its resistance.

The SI unit of resistance is the ohm (symbol Ω – the Greek letter
omega).

A conductor's resistance can be considered in two ways:

(1) as a mathematical constant, relating the current through a
     conductor to the potential difference applied across it (as
     expressed in Ohm's law); or
(2) as a physical feature, depending principally on three features:
     (i) its length, (ii) its cross-sectional area, and (iii) the resistivity
     of the material of which the conductor is made – i.e. the
     property that quantifies its opposition to electron flow, in
     specific circumstances. So, if a conductor's cross-sectional
     area is reduced, its resistance increases, reducing the current
     that will flow in response to the application of a given poten-
     tial difference.

Inherent filtration

This is the filtration of the X-ray beam due to the X-ray tube components through which the photons pass while travelling from the
tube target as far as the tube window: superficial layers of the target,
the envelope wall, oil, and the window itself.

Added filtration

This is a thin plate of aluminium installed across the tube port, to
supplement the tube's inherent filtration.

Cooling paths

Cooling of the focal track occurs almost immediately after the start of an exposure, when the area that has been the first to act as the target moves away, into an unheated position. From the focal track, heat is conducted to the body of the disc. The efficiency of this process relates directly to the area of the focal track's interface with the remainder of the disc, both along its (circular) length and at its internal and external perimeters. These increase in proportion to the disc's diameter. A large temperature difference – a steep **temperature gradient** – also encourages heat conduction from the focal track to the body of the disc, so any feature that increases the disc's thermal capacity will make conduction occur more rapidly.

The role of the stem

The stem on which the disc is mounted has a small cross-sectional area. This appears to be a strange design feature, since it forms only a skeletal link from the disc across to the anode's rotor, and suggests poor mechanical stability. But the anode stem is made from molybdenum, which is a very strong metal, and its thin design is justified by its effect on how heat losses occur. The stem's narrowness reduces harmful heat conduction from the disc towards the anode's rotation mechanism. In doing this, it tends to sustain the disc's high temperature, maintaining a relatively high temperature gradient between the disc and its surroundings, boosting heat loss by radiation (the intended, safe and efficient method).

Loss of efficiency through ageing

As it ages, an X-ray tube will naturally begin to show signs of wear. These changes, which can reduce the tube's efficiency, may be irreversible because, unlike some other items of equipment, direct maintenance is normally impossible: the insert is a sealed unit. But some limited forms of compensation can be achieved: by re-adjusting the voltages supplied by the generator or modifying X-ray exposure factors.

At the cathode

Despite being small, X-ray tube filaments are strong (sometimes described as 'rugged') and good at withstanding the stresses of repeated use. But gradually, the filament wire becomes thinner:

Two

vaporisation of tungsten from its heated surface leaves a filament unable to emit electrons at the required rate for delivering a selected tube current. This form of deterioration is detected, and corrective adjustments are made, when X-ray equipment undergoes its regular service inspections. The thinning of a tube's filaments (broad and fine) increases their **electrical resistance**. To compensate, the filament voltages supplied by the generator are increased slightly, raising the heating currents, so that correct rates of thermionic emission are restored. Because this modification raises the filaments' operating temperatures, the rate of vaporisation unfortunately also increases, but X-ray production rates are sustained for a period, and the tube's useful service is extended.

Some of the vaporised tungsten becomes deposited on the inner surface of the envelope wall. As the tube ages, this deposit becomes thicker, tending, because of tungsten's high atomic number, to increase the tube's **inherent filtration** and (by absorption) reduce beam intensity.

At the anode

An X-ray tube's efficiency in converting filament electrons' kinetic energy to X-ray energy is at its maximum when the tube is new. The surface of the focal track is smooth, so the high-speed electrons tend to penetrate to an even depth. This is significant because in order to contribute to the X-ray beam, photons must first emerge through the target's superficial layers. Although these are relatively thin, a fraction of the X-ray energy is absorbed before it can be used. This limits the beam's intensity – but it is a normal effect for which no compensation is required.

When a tungsten disc has been in use for a period of time, the focal track may begin to suffer the effects of repeated heating and cooling. Internal tensions can make the metal brittle, roughening its surface, so that a network of fine cracks develops. When exposures are made, some filament electrons can then enter the cracks, penetrating deeper into the anode, increasing the average depth at which X-ray production occurs. The effect of this change becomes gradually apparent in practice, as a reduction in the X-ray beam's intensity. To compensate, electrical energy is applied to the tube at a higher rate (by raising kV or mA) and exposure times may be lengthened. But this is only a temporary solution because, unlike X-ray production, conversion of the electrons' kinetic energy into *heat* is not affected. The increased exposure factors produce even more heat, in proportion to the X-ray output, so the damage continues to occur.

Tungsten's tendency to become brittle is markedly reduced when it is alloyed with another metal, *rhenium*, typically in the ratio 90% tungsten: 10% rhenium. The use of rhenium does not reduce the focal track's ability to produce X-rays: while its melting point is 200° lower than tungsten's, its atomic number is actually higher (75, compared with 74) so energy conversion efficiency is maintained.

X-ray tube manufacturers have occasionally tried out other features of disc design to cope with the effects of heat production. For example, expansion grooves can be moulded along the inner and outer perimeters of the focal track, and radial slots formed, to divide the circular disc area into free-edged segments. Both these features can minimise thermal stresses: the grooves and slots accommodate the expansion that occurs when the focal track's temperature rises.

The thin stem on which the disc is mounted has already been mentioned as a factor in boosting the disc's cooling rate. Its other effect – restricting heat conduction towards the anode's rotation mechanism – provides protection against premature wear. When its temperature rises, the all-metal rotor mechanism tends to expand, narrowing the clearances between its moving parts. This puts extra pressure on its bearings, grinding their surfaces and reducing their efficiency. So, rotational speed tends to reduce over a period of time, potentially causing further thermal damage to the focal track.

Safety issues involved in X-ray production and control

Introduction

Exposure to ionising radiations potentially presents a risk to the patient. X-ray examinations go ahead – i.e. they are justified – if potential risks are outweighed by expected benefits. But these judgements are based on an assumption that the X-ray equipment is functioning correctly. Equipment is built to high standards and incorporates safety features; legislation effectively forbids the sale of unsafe equipment.

But in practice, safety can be assumed only if the equipment is

▪ used correctly by fully-trained staff, following manufacturers' instructions, and in accordance with current safety legislation;
▪ covered by a rigorous quality assurance programme, ensuring that dangerous conditions never develop.

Radiation hazards command prime consideration but the nature of X-ray equipment is such that there are also potential electrical and

Total filtration

This is the sum of inherent and added filtration, which must meet the value stipulated by prevailing radiation protection regulations – e.g. 2.5 mm or 3.0 mm aluminium (equivalent).

Aluminium equivalent

Only (pure) aluminium sheet can be specified as a 'thickness of aluminium'. The filtration of X-ray photons by other materials, e.g. glass and oil, is measured in terms of 'aluminium equivalent' – i.e. the thickness of aluminium sheet that would have the same filtration effect.

(There is a similarity to the practice of using 'lead equivalent' as a means of measuring the effectiveness (as an X-ray attenuator) of a protective barrier composed of other materials instead of, or in addition to, lead.)

Interlocks

An interlock is a device that links two or more functions together, to ensure that they take place safely in a correct order. An everyday example is found in a microwave oven or a tumble dryer: an electrical switch operated by the door ensures that it must be firmly closed before the appliance will operate. X-ray equipment interlocks usually concern physical or radiation safety.

Others are designed to protect the X-ray tube, allowing or preventing an X-ray exposure, depending on the tube's readiness.

Circuit breakers

Electrical components and conductors have their safety 'rated' in terms of the maximum safe currents they are allowed to conduct. Provided that the current does not rise above the rated value, heat generation will not cause a dangerous temperature rise: conditions will remain safe; e.g. insulation will remain intact.

Circuit breakers, like fuses, are designed as 'weak links' within a circuit. If a current exceeds its rated maximum value, the increased magnetic effect will operate a circuit breaker's 'off' switch by pulling

physical or mechanical dangers; and it must be recognised that both staff and patients require protection.

Radiation safety

Leakage radiation

X-radiation is emitted from the tube target in all directions but it is important that X-ray emission from the tube should be confined to its window (and then be controlled further by collimation). The sheet lead that lines the tube housing provides appropriate protection: it efficiently absorbs X-rays emitted from the target in 'other' directions, so that leakage intensity from the tube housing is insignificantly low, within the permitted limit.

Low-energy photons: beam quality and filtration

X-ray exposures would be less harmful if every photon emerging from the X-ray tube could contribute to forming the image. This condition cannot be met: the X-ray beam is heterogeneous; it contains a range of braking radiation photon energies and some low-energy characteristic photons. Some photon energies are so low that the photons are incapable of reaching the image receptor, even if their paths lie through the most radiolucent parts of the patient's body. Such photons contribute nothing to image formation. Instead – and worse – they increase the biological risks to the patient. These hazards are minimised by beam filtration.

While still inside the X-ray tube, crossing the short distance between where they are produced within the target and the window, photons encounter absorbing layers formed by the tube's components: the target itself, the envelope wall, oil, and window seal. This inherent filtration prevents a proportion of low energy photons from leaving the tube. But it normally fails to meet the minimum level of **total** filtration stipulated by radiation protection regulations, and needs to be supplemented by **added filtration**. This takes the form of a metal plate permanently fitted across the tube's port. Its radiopacity is relatively low: while removing low-energy photons from the beam, it must also allow relatively free transmission of high-energy photons. Choice of filter material and thickness is determined by radiation quality. For diagnostic X-rays, aluminium (atomic number 13) is suitably radiopaque. Its thickness, typically in the range 1.5 mm to 3 mm is directly measurable, while inherent filtration is measured in terms of its **aluminium equivalent**.

Two

Prevention of accidental exposures

Precautions are built into an X-ray generator to prevent X-ray exposures from being made accidentally or prematurely. **Interlocks** link and monitor functions, to ensure safety. A generator's exposure switch must be designed so that only deliberate effort (not accidental pressure) will trigger an exposure. If left unattended for a period of time, an X-ray generator should be switched off and locked, to prevent malicious misuse.

Prevention of accidental exposure involves not only the equipment itself but also the area in which it operates. Permanent installations must be planned and built in such a way that protective barriers and warning signs guarantee the safety of all personnel when exposures are being (and are about to be) made.

Electrical safety

In their design and construction, all items of X-ray equipment must conform to strict electrical safety regulations, both to protect personnel and to prevent damage to the equipment itself. They must be used with care, and regularly inspected to ensure that vulnerable external features (cables, flexes and sockets) are undamaged and show no signs of wear. If any malfunction is suspected, this must be reported immediately and the equipment taken out of service until it has been thoroughly checked, repaired and declared safe. Safety must be maintained at the highest level, without compromise. *Unsafe equipment must never be used.*

Shockproofing

Some safety measures are found in all electrical apparatus and installations: emergency **circuit breakers** or fuses are incorporated to prevent currents rising to dangerously high values, and circuits are insulated to prevent leakage of charge. If insulation fails, electric charge tends to seek out a path to zero potential, usually termed 'earth' or 'ground'. Serious, potentially fatal electrical accidents occur when this path to earth involves a person's body. Where high voltages (arbitrarily, in excess of 1000 V) are involved, another feature is provided to give extra protection: insulation is surrounded by a metallic shield at earth potential. If insulation fails, the leaking charge has an immediate, low resistance path to earth without endangering persons who may be touching or close to the equipment. For obvious reasons, this provision is known as **shockproofing**.

Components in the X-ray high-voltage circuit (i.e. high-voltage and tube-filament transformers, high-voltage rectifiers, cables linking the generator to the X-ray tube, and the tube itself) are shockproofed. X-ray tubes and high-voltage transformers are situated within metallic, shockproofed tanks at earth potential. The tank cavities are filled with an insulating liquid, a special, non-degradable mineral oil. This fills every part of the cavity more effectively than a solid, excluding air and also acting as a convectant, carrying heat to the outer (cooler) walls.

Tube filament transformers (only) provide the low voltages required for heating the tube filaments; but because of their connections to the high-voltage cathode, they too must be situated within the shockproofed tank. High-frequency technology, which has increased transformer efficiency, and improved rectifier design now enable X-ray generators to be considerably smaller than their older, low-frequency counterparts. Size may be reduced so much as to allow the high-voltage circuit to be included with the X-ray tube insert, in a single, extended housing. Otherwise, the high-voltage link between generator and X-ray tube is provided by special high-voltage cables. These incorporate high-efficiency, flexible insulation, surrounded by equally flexible woven metal braiding. This forms an unbroken, earthed connection between the tube's housing and the high-voltage transformer tank, to shockproof the cables. The braiding is protected against abrasive damage by an outer, easily cleaned, plastic sleeve. See Figure 2.1.

Safety at the control panel

Electrical protection for staff who operate X-ray equipment is ensured by circuit design as well as general safety features. Both the high-tension and the tube filament transformers have fixed **turns ratios**, so their output voltages are related to their inputs by constant factors. So, the transformers' effects (on kilovoltage and tube filament temperature) are controlled by adjustment of their input voltages. This arrangement offers built-in safety. Because there is no electrical conducting path across from a transformer's primary to its secondary winding, there is no risk of extending the X-ray tube's high voltage dangers to the kV and mA selectors mounted on the control panel.

An exposure indicator on the X-ray generator's control panel is activated during every exposure. The only way that this can operate reliably is by receiving or sampling the actual X-ray tube current.

a connecting bar away from its terminals. (Fuses operate through the current's increased heating effect, raising the fuse's temperature, causing it to melt and break the circuit.) The re-setting of a circuit breaker is much quicker than replacing a fuse – a convenience that, in some circumstances, can have safety implications.

Shockproof

The insulation of electrical conductors is a standard safety precaution. Most electrical appliances also feature an earth connection – to a conductor that (eventually) terminates literally in the earth. This provides a universal escape route for any leaking electric charge (positive or negative) preventing it from accumulating, or seeking a path to earth through the body of anyone who touches it.

Equipment such as an X-ray tube, operating at a high voltage is shockproofed by the enclosure of its insulation within a metallic, earthed shell. In the event of insulation failure, charge passes directly to earth, without posing a life-threatening hazard to a person who touches the faulty equipment.

Turns ratio

The turns ratio indicates the relative number of turns around the core, of a transformer's primary and secondary windings. This establishes the ratio between the input and output voltages, according to whether the device is intended to increase ('step-up') or reduce ('step-down') the applied voltage. Most transformers have a fixed turns ratio. So, whatever input voltage is applied across its primary winding, a predictable output voltage will be induced across its secondary winding. This arrangement means that the transformer's output voltage can only be varied by a proportionate change in its input voltage. An X-ray generator's high-voltage transformer and filament transformer both operate on this basis.

Counterbalancing

Heavy items of equipment, such as a X-ray tubes, which must be moved carefully and precisely during the course of their use, are mounted in such a way that a permanent upward force acts on them,

This appears difficult, because of the tube's high-voltage operation. But a safe connection to the high-voltage circuit is possible: at the mid-point of the high-voltage transformer's secondary winding, which is at earth potential, to balance the electrical stresses across the circuit.

Physical and mechanical safety

All X-ray equipment is expensive; some of it is large and heavy. When moved around, there is a risk of physical damage, so it must always be handled carefully. For very heavy items, **counterbalancing** is essential, and power-assistance is helpful, especially when coupled with pressure-sensitive switches, to switch off the driving force if equipment gets too close to an obstacle. Mobile units and installations in 24-hour emergency rooms may tend to be more at risk than others, but all equipment should receive regular mechanical checks, covering brakes, locks, weight-bearing supports and cables. X-ray tubes are moved around constantly, and contain a vulnerable evacuated insert, so they require particular care. Protection features of tube construction include the following.

Oil expansion

The insulating/convecting oil, sealed within the housing's cavity, could be a source of damage. When the tube is in use, the oil's temperature rises, making it expand and potentially exert increased pressure both on the evacuated insert and the walls of the housing. To ensure safety, the cavity's wall incorporates a flexible diaphragm that moves in and out, as the oil's volume changes, preventing pressure from increasing. Situated directly outside the diaphragm is a sensitive switch that will be operated if expansion should ever reach a danger threshold. If this occurs, the tube's electrical supplies are disconnected, enforcing a cooling-off period, before the tube can be used again.

The tube envelope

Conventional X-ray tube envelopes are made from special, heat-resistant, borosilicate glass, very similar to the type used for kitchen ovenware. Sudden rises in temperature, with exposure to high levels of radiant heat, are tolerated without strain. In addition, this type of glass is strong, radiolucent and a good electrical insulator.

Two

exactly equalling and opposing the downward force caused by gravity. This arrangement effectively makes the equipment 'weightless', preventing it from posing a danger (it cannot fall) and allowing easy adjustment of its position.

Incandescence

Emission of light as a result of being heated to a high temperature.

Vaporisation

This term describes the change from a solid or liquid state into a vapour that occurs when a solid or liquid is heated. Within an X-ray tube, the heat produced during its operation causes tungsten atoms to be lost from the anode and filament surfaces, into the surrounding vacuum. The surface of the anode becomes eroded and, more significantly, the filaments become thinner.

This process must not be confused with thermionic emission – the emission of electrons.

X-ray tube 'preparation'

To protect it from unnecessary and premature wear, an X-ray tube is kept in a stand-by mode until just before an exposure is to be made. Each exposure is preceded by a brief 'preparation', satisfying two needs:

(1) the anode is set in motion and allowed time to reach its full rotational speed; and

(2) the filament is boosted from its stand-by temperature, up to the full operational temperature, appropriate to the selected tube current.

Controlled area

This term is used generally in safety legislation to indicate an area where there are inherent dangers; admission is allowed only to authorised persons. In the context of radiation protection, this term

The tube filaments

(a) To achieve the required rates of thermionic emission, the filaments operate at very high temperatures. They are heated to a state of **incandescence**, which also raises the rate of **vaporisation**: atoms of tungsten leave the filament wire, reducing its cross-sectional area, and forming a deposit on the inner wall of the tube insert. This has already been mentioned as a potential factor in reducing efficiency but it may also pose a threat to safety. A heavy tungsten deposit on a glass envelope forms an isolated, conducting area on which electric charge can accumulate, creating a risk of discharge, which could damage the glass wall, destroy the vacuum and bring the tube's operation to an abrupt end. So, the filament is only raised to its full emission temperature just before an exposure is made – as part of the tube's **preparation** (Figure 2.21).

(b) A filament – particularly one already weakened by vaporisation – could be fractured by the shock of suddenly being heated from 'cold' (room temperature) up to its high, operating temperature, just before an exposure is made. The risk of such damage is reduced by keeping the filament at a heated, stand-by level, a step below its operating temperature. This is sufficiently low to avoid significant vaporisation but high enough to reduce the interval through which the filament temperature has to be raised during the tube preparation phase. After each exposure, the filament automatically reverts to its stand-by temperature until boosted again, in preparation for the next.

The anode disc

Thermal shock can also cause stress damage to the anode disc at the start of a working period, when there could be a sudden change from 'cold' to a high temperature. Focal tracks made of a tungsten–rhenium alloy withstand stress better than pure tungsten, but further protection can be achieved by employing a sequence of low-factor 'warm-up' exposures. These are recommended before a tube anode is subjected to the full impact of the first, image-producing exposures of the working day. The exposures generate gentle heat pulses, taking the focal track through a small, gradual temperature rise. This procedure produces X-rays (although for no purpose) so the tube diaphragms must be firmly closed beforehand and normal radiation protection precautions must be observed: no-one is allowed within the **controlled area**. Following the warm-up period,

describes the area immediately surrounding the patient and the X-ray tube while an exposure is being made, where the radiation intensity (or the absorbed dose rate) is sufficiently high to cause biological harm. The area comprises two parts:

(1) the entire path of the primary beam continuing beyond the patient and image receptor until it encounters a protective barrier, appropriate to the radiation energy, e.g. for X-radiation, a brick or concrete wall or a lead screen;

(2) an imaginary sphere, centred on the patient, within which the intensity of the scattered radiation remains hazardous. The dimensions of this sphere are related to the tube kilovoltage (which controls photon energy): a radius of 2 metres covers most circumstances but a safety margin may be added as a further precaution.

Normally, the patient is the only person allowed to remain within the controlled area. If anyone else attends, such as a relative who is giving support or reassurance to a nervous patient, written consent must be given and the circumstances must be fully documented.

Anode lubrication

Rotation of the anode cannot be lubricated by oil-based compounds: they vaporise at high temperatures and would contaminate the vacuum within the insert, causing the tube to malfunction. Instead, lubrication is achieved by use of appropriate metals – e.g. silver – that resist vaporisation and remain effective, even at high temperatures.

Stator windings

An ordinary electric motor comprises a rotational mechanism, immediately surrounded by coils that produce the magnetic fields required for rotation. In the case of an X-ray tube, the inner part, the anode's *rotor*, lies within the evacuated envelope. The coils that induce its rotation, the *stator windings*, are positioned outside the envelope, aligned closely to the rotor, to ensure efficiency. Separation simplifies electrical connections and does not threaten the integrity of the vacuum.

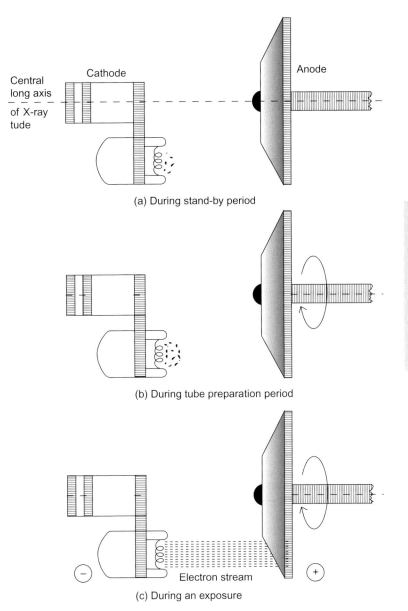

Figure 2.21 X-ray tube preparation. (a) During stand-by periods, between expo-sures, the filament is maintained at a low temperature, with little activity, and no rotational force is applied to the anode. (b) When the tube is prepared for an expo-sure, the filament temperature is boosted to produce the rate of thermionic emis-sion, and the anode is set in motion. (c) During exposures, the selected kilovoltage is applied between the cathode and anode, creating the tube current. The elec-trons bombard a focal track, moving at full speed.

Resonance

This phenomenon occurs when a structure is exposed to potentially dangerous vibrational energy of a wavelength that coincides (either exactly or in multiple units) with its dimensions, particularly at high intensities.

the anode temperature is kept sufficiently high by the heat arising from routine use.

Anode rotation mechanism

Tube preparation triggers anode rotation and imposes a short delay, allowing time for acceleration up to the full speed. The anode rotation mechanism is specially **lubricated** during manufacture but eventually the bearings show signs of wear, with rotation becoming slower and noisier. Over-prolonged rotation causes unnecessary wear, so tube preparation should be withheld until just before an exposure is required. Normally, following an exposure, the driving voltage is completely removed from the **stator windings**, leaving the anode to slow to a halt. But high-speed anode rotation can present additional problems: vibration may occur at certain frequencies, as the anode slows down, causing harmful **resonance**. To avoid this, a braking voltage is applied, rapidly reducing the rotational speed, minimising the risk of damage.

Two

Chapter 3
Formation of the emergent beam

Introduction

It is popularly known that 'X-rays pass through the body' but it is essential also to recognise that *some do not*. Expressed in radiographic terms: when an object is exposed to a diagnostic X-ray beam,

- some X-ray photons are **transmitted** – they penetrate the object and reach the image receptor;
- other photons are **attenuated** – they fail to reach the image receptor because, while passing through the object, they have been removed from the X-ray beam.

The beam emerging from an object carries a pattern of varying X-ray intensities, showing where and to what extent transmission and attenuation have occurred. The variations are due primarily to the object's composition – its mixture of **radiopaque** and **radiolucent** parts – but they are also strongly influenced by the X-ray beam's quality.

This chapter outlines the two principal attenuation processes involved in X-ray image formation, and how their occurrence varies with both the object's composition and the beam's quality. The practical significance of these attenuation processes is then considered: their influence on image quality and radiation protection.

X-ray attenuation processes

Attenuation of a diagnostic X-ray beam is due to the combined, simultaneous effects of **absorption** and **scattering** (Figure 3.1).

X-ray transmission

Transmitted X-ray photons are those that pass through the object without being involved in an interaction. They form the emergent beam, indicating areas of radiolucency within the object.

X-ray attenuation

This is an overall term, used to indicate *removal of energy from the X-ray beam* by either absorption or scattering.

Radiopacity and radiolucency

These terms indicate the difficulty or ease with which a structure is penetrated by X-ray photons. A *radiolucent* structure tends to allow X-ray photons to be transmitted through it; *radiopaque* indicates that it tends to attenuate X-rays. Practically all substances show a degree of both radiolucency and radiopacity, so these terms may be used relatively.

X-ray absorption

This is defined as the transfer of energy from an X-ray beam to an irradiated structure.

Scattering

Scattering is the process by which X-ray photons interact with matter, then change their direction of travel. In diagnostic radiography, the change of direction presents two problems. First, it makes the photons unable to represent any information about the structure with which they have interacted – so if their energy is eventually absorbed by the image receptor, it cannot contribute to image formation. Second, scattered photons present an uncontrolled danger to tissues lying outside the area of the body that is being shown on the image. The patient is primarily at risk – particularly if these other tissues have greater sensitivity to the effects of radiation – but the hazard will also extend outside the patient's body. This

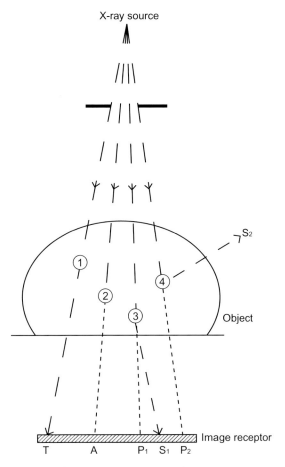

X-ray source

S₂

Object

Image receptor

T   A   P₁ S₁ P₂

Figure 3.1 Summary of the processes occurring during an X-ray exposure. Photon 1 is *transmitted* through the object, unchanged until its energy is absorbed by the image receptor (at T), contributing *by exposure* to the formation of the latent image. Photon 2 is *photoelectrically absorbed*: it disappears, transferring its energy to the object. The area of the image receptor aligned to its path (A) receives no exposure (from this photon) – so, by default, a point of *non-exposure* is contributed to the latent image, complementing the effects of the transmitted photons. Photon 3 undergoes a *Compton interaction*. After losing part of its energy by absorption, the photon is *scattered*: its path changes, causing an approach to the image receptor at a different angle. Non-exposure of the point aligned to its original path (P₁) contributes evidence of *absorption* to the image, but scattering prevents the photon from contributing further information about the object. The scattered photon's absorption by the image receptor at (S₁) imposes noise on the image signal, and tends (combined with other scattered photons) to *reduce the image's contrast*. Photon 4 also undergoes a *Compton interaction* and, like photon 3, it contributes *evidence of absorption* to the image (by its non-exposure of P₂). This photon's scattering angle takes it away from the image receptor, so it does not reduce image contrast. Instead, it poses a *potential radiation hazard* in the area (S₂) surrounding the object.

Three

There are two distinct interactions: *photoelectric absorption* and the *Compton process*. Both cause removal of electrons from atoms within the object; in other words, **ionisation**.

Photoelectric absorption

The photoelectric absorption process happens when an X-ray photon collides with an inner-shell electron, 'firmly bound' by attraction to its atom's nucleus, provided that the photon's energy equals or exceeds the electron's **binding energy** (Figure 3.2).

(1)   The collision removes the electron from its shell. This action transfers some of the photon's energy to the atom. Any remaining energy (original photon energy *minus* binding energy) is given to the displaced electron, as its kinetic energy. With this acquired energy, the electron, now termed a photo-electron, leaves the atom – which temporarily becomes a positive ion.

(2)   An electron from a shell further away from the nucleus fills the shell vacancy left by the photoelectron. As it travels inwards, this electron loses energy until, when the transition is complete and the vacancy has been filled, it has lost pre-cisely the difference between the binding energies of the two shells – the one that it left and the one that it joined. This is emitted as a photon of characteristic electromagnetic energy (*not* X-rays).

(3)   The transition creates a vacancy in the outer shell. This is filled by an electron from a shell even further out; and any other consequent vacancies are similarly filled, until ionisation has been reversed – i.e. until the positive ion becomes a neutral atom again.

When these stages are complete, the atom has re-emitted the energy it originally acquired from the photon.

   To summarise: this is a process of complete absorption: the photon's energy is converted into:

▨   the photoelectron's kinetic energy, and
▨   the characteristic radiation emitted by the atom.

This energy is absorbed within surrounding cells, so there is a complete transfer of the X-ray photon's energy to the exposed tissue.

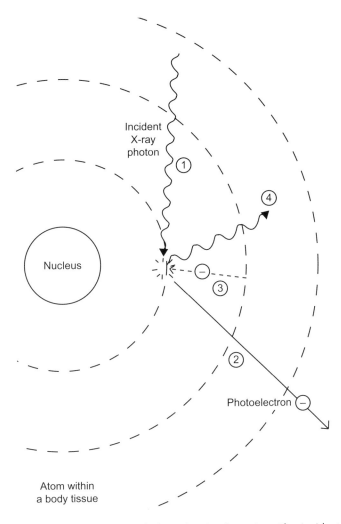

Figure 3.2 Schematic diagram of photoelectric absorption. The incident X-ray photon 1 collides with a firmly-bound, inner-shell electron 2, ejecting it from the atom, as a photoelectron. The inner-shell vacancy is filled by the transition of an electron 3 from an outer shell, accompanied by the emission of a photon of characteristic radiation, 4.

The Compton process

The Compton process may occur when an X-ray photon collides with a 'free', outer-shell electron, only loosely bound and distant from its atom's nucleus (Figure 3.3). This collision has two outcomes.

Three

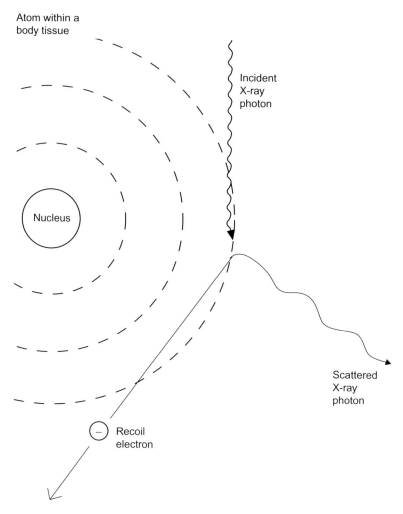

Figure 3.3 Schematic diagram of the Compton process. The incident X-ray photon collides with a loosely-bound, outer-shell electron. The electron 'recoils' from the collision with acquired kinetic energy, while the photon is scattered and follows an altered path, with reduced energy.

(1) The outer-shell electron gains some energy from the photon, as kinetic energy, and leaves the site of the collision. It is said to 'recoil', becoming a *recoil electron* – also known as a *Compton electron*.

(2) The X-ray photon, retaining the remainder of its former energy, changes course: it scatters – i.e. it no longer travels along a straight line traceable back to the X-ray tube target. Instead, it follows a different path, still in a straight line but now in a random direction. The angle through which a photon

scatters is related to its original energy and to the energy it loses.

Recoil electrons are absorbed within surrounding cells, as are *some* of the scattered photons, so this process comprises scattering and partial absorption.

The influence of types of body tissue

Photoelectric absorption

Photoelectric absorption tends mostly to occur in areas of the body where 'firmly-bound' electrons are relatively plentiful. Electrons' binding energies are directly related to the positive charge on the atom's nucleus – i.e. they increase with atomic number. So, photoelectric absorption occurs principally in tissues that have a high **effective atomic number**. The natural sites are skeletal: bone, containing calcium (atomic number 20) has an effective atomic number of approximately 14. Absorption also occurs significantly when photons collide with molecules of opaque contrast agents, containing either barium (atomic number 56) or iodine (53).

The fraction of energy removed from an X-ray beam by photoelectric absorption when it passes through a body tissue or other medium, is directly proportional to *the cubed value* of its effective atomic number.

The Compton process

The fraction of energy removed from an X-ray beam by the Compton process is directly proportional to the object's **electron density** – i.e. the Compton process tends to occur in body structures where there is a high concentration of electrons per unit mass. The chemical element with a particularly high electron density is hydrogen, which is abundant in the body as a constituent of water and fat. So, the Compton process is primarily responsible for X-ray attenuation in soft tissue areas of the body.

The influence of beam quality

As well as studying how the body's various structures and tissues affect attenuation processes, it is important to see what happens

Three

underlies the concept of a *controlled area*, and explains the wide-spread use of protective screens.

Ionisation

An atom is electrically neutral: it contains equal numbers of positive charges (protons, within the nucleus) and negative charges (electrons arranged in the shells). Removal of a charge destroys the balance: it converts the atom into an ion. This process is termed ionisation. So, when an atom loses an electron, it becomes a positively-charged ion. The freed electron is a negative ion. Molecules (bonded groups of atoms) can be significantly changed by ionisation.

Shell binding energy

Electrons orbiting the atom's nucleus are held within their shells by the force of attraction (positive acting on negative) exerted by the nucleus. These forces are stronger for elements with higher atomic numbers, and are inversely related to the square of the distance between a shell and the nucleus – i.e. acting more strongly on electrons nearer the nucleus. A shell's binding energy is defined as the energy required to remove one of its electrons. Binding energies are higher for inner shells than for those further away from the nucleus. Each element has a unique, characteristic set of binding energies.

Effective atomic number

An element has an atomic number. A pure substance, composed of a single element, reacts – e.g. in the photoelectric absorption of X-rays – according to this atomic number. A substance composed of two or more elements reacts in these circumstances according to an average that takes into account both the atomic numbers of the constituent elements and the relative proportions in which the elements are combined. This is termed the *effective* atomic number.

Electron density

This term indicates the number of electrons present within a unit mass of a substance or material.

It is tempting to make the false assumption that electron density rises with atomic number, because the higher the atomic number, the greater the number of electrons in each atom. This overlooks the fact that atoms become more massive as the atomic number increases: both protons and neutrons are added to the nucleus. Owing to this, the ratio between an element's atomic number and the number of electrons per atom is fairly constant for all elements – and for this reason, the fraction of energy removed from an X-ray beam by the Compton process is described as being *independent of atomic number*.

But there is an exceptional element: hydrogen. Its unique status is explained by considering the role of the neutron – the nuclear particle that carries no electric charge. Put simply, its purpose is to keep the protons together. Otherwise, mutual repulsion would separate them. The hydrogen nucleus comprises a single proton; there is no need of a neutron. So, the nucleus has a mass of 1, forming a 1:1 ratio with its single, orbiting electron.

The contrast between hydrogen and other elements is simply illustrated by considering helium (atomic number 2). Each helium atom has two electrons *but* its nucleus comprises two protons and two neutrons – so its mass is four; the ratio of *electrons to mass* is 1:2. In other words, helium's electron density is only half that of hydrogen.

Hydrogen is most abundant in the body as a constituent of water and fat. Compton attenuation is proportionally higher in these substances and their tissues.

Commentary

Relative and absolute

'Relative' compares what is being described with other, similar substances, properties or phenomena, either by statement or implication.

'Absolute' indicates that the described features are considered or judged on their own, with reference to nothing but baseline criteria. For example, the Kelvin temperature scale measures zero in a situation at which all atomic vibration is considered to have ceased. It was formerly known as the absolute zero temperature (= minus 273 degrees Celsius).

when X-ray beam quality changes. In practice, this means considering how X-ray attenuation can be controlled by the selected tube kilovoltage.

Photoelectric absorption

When kV is increased, occurrence of photoelectric absorption (which depends on photons interacting with *firmly-bound* electrons) undergoes a steep reduction. This happens because, as photon energies increase, there is a fall in the number of 'firmly bound' electrons. There is no actual change in the electrons' binding energies: these are fixed properties of the shells, and determined by an element's atomic number. But the label 'firmly' is **relative**, rather then **absolute**. An electron may indeed be 'firmly bound' if a *low-energy* photon collides with it, but it tends to lose this status when in collision with a photon of higher energy.

So, as kilovoltage increases and fewer 'firmly bound' electrons are available, the fraction of energy absorbed from the beam reduces: approximately in proportion to the *cubed value of the tube kilovoltage*.

The Compton process

When kV is increased, there is also a reduction in the fraction of energy absorbed and scattered from the beam by the Compton process. This can be explained as an effect of increased penetration: as photon energies increase, collisions with free electrons become less significant.

There is a simple **inverse** relationship (not as marked as in the case of photoelectric absorption): the fraction of energy removed from the beam by the Compton process is *inversely proportional to tube kilovoltage*.

Practical relevance

A study of X-ray attenuation processes is fundamental to understanding both image quality and radiation protection, when factors are being selected for exposing a radiographic image. The appropriate *quantity* of X-ray energy for each image, taking into account the object's overall mass, the focus–image distance, the speed of the image receptor, etc., can be ensured by the use of an automatic

Three

exposure device (AED). But selection of the beam's *quality* – i.e. the tube kilovoltage – requires a closer evaluation of the object.

The object's radiopacity acts as a guide to the beam penetration required; photons must penetrate the object sufficiently to record an image. But if penetration were the only purpose underlying kV selection, it would be logical and labour-saving to set the generator to produce a standard, high kV value for every image, on the basis that penetration could always be guaranteed. Instead, a kV value is individually selected for each exposure – normally, to match the most radiopaque part of the object required for showing full diagnostic information. Before an exposure is made, it may be difficult to predict how much X-ray energy the object will remove from the X-ray beam, *as an absolute amount*. But it is normally possible to anticipate *the fractions of energy* that will be absorbed and scattered by the object, and how these fractions will vary with changes in kV. Two principal issues underlie kV selection, in addition to achieving penetration of the object: *image contrast* and *radiation protection*.

Kilovoltage selection and image contrast

In an imaging department, the kilovoltages required for most radiographic projections are well established: ranges, if not precise values, have been identified and can normally be used with confidence. But there are occasions when, perhaps owing to the patient's build or a suspected pathology, an area of the body varies from the usual 'standard', and some kV readjustment is required. As a rule, *over*estimation of kV values – i.e. selection of values higher than actually required – is judged to be safer than *under*estimation, because this avoids the problem of under-penetration. But overestimation must be accompanied by awareness of the contrast reduction that is likely to occur.

Contrast due to absorption

X-ray absorption occurs owing to a combination of the photoelectric and Compton processes. Concerning, first, areas of the body where the two processes tend to occur evenly: an increase in beam quality (kV) raises penetration; overall, the object absorbs a smaller fraction of the incident beam's energy. It is important to recognise that when this occurs, there is a reduction in *the differences between* the fractions absorbed by the various parts of the object. So, the

Three

Direct and inverse relationships

These terms are paired to describe scientific or mathematical relationships, between properties when their values either increase or reduce. Two properties are *directly* linked when they both increase (or reduce) together, at an identified rate. An *inverse* relationship exists where, as one property increases, the other reduces, and vice versa.

'High kV'

This term describes a radiographic procedure where the chosen tube kilovoltage is high, not only to ensure penetration of the object but beyond this, to reduce image contrast (owing to the weakening effect of photoelectric absorption). This is a *deliberate* reduction of image contrast, for the purpose of increasing the image's diagnostic value – most commonly when the chest is examined. This effect must not be confused with *accidental* contrast reduction resulting from, for example, a failure to exclude the effect of scatter or the failure to maintain image processing QA standards; these *reduce* diagnostic value.

Exponential relationships

Two properties are said to be related exponentially if equal *amounts* of one are related to equal *fractions* (*percentages*) of the other (Figure 3.5).

Exponential relationships can affect increasing values – where the phenomenon is known as growth – or their reduction, also termed decay. The following examples illustrate this phenomenon and its significance.

Radioactive elements (as covered in Chapter 6) lose their radioactivity by a process of exponential decay. As each equal period of time passes, activity reduces by an identified fraction or percentage. For convenience, the time taken for a *50%* reduction in activity is commonly identified – known as the 'half life'. Environmental concern for safety in the vicinity of radioactive waste deposits arises from a consequence of the exponential 'law': the nature of this reduction – e.g. by halving – means that a zero figure can never be reached.

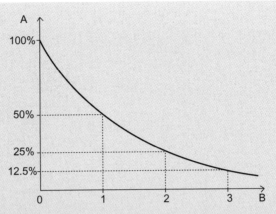

Figure 3.5 Exponential decay. Property A reduces by a fixed percentage, for each unit quantity of Property B. This graph shows the first part of the decay – which continues with A becoming progressively smaller but never reaching zero. Examples of A / B: radioactivity / time, and X-ray intensity / barrier thickness.

Attenuation of diagnostic X-rays tends primarily to be considered in the context of image formation – particularly concerning image contrast. But attenuation is also the purpose of protective barriers, whether based on the use of lead or some other appropriate material. Barriers, such as the protective screen that surrounds an X-ray generator's control panel, or the lead sheet that lines an X-ray tube's housing, reduce X-ray intensity exponentially.

Incremental increase of a barrier's thickness increases it effectiveness but, as shown by the previous example, radiation intensity can never be reduced to zero. This should not provoke alarm, because the minimum to which a barrier reduces radiation intensity is calculated to be safe, provided that specified conditions are met, including limits on:

- the intensity of the incident radiation (effectively, how close the barrier is to its source);
- the radiation quality (effectively, the tube kV);
- how closely personnel are situated beyond the barrier;
- the time for which personnel occupy positions beyond the barrier.

Every barrier bears a plate or label, displaying its composition, expressed either in millimetres of lead or (in the case of clothing or lead glass) *lead equivalent* (i.e. to match its effect).

Commentary

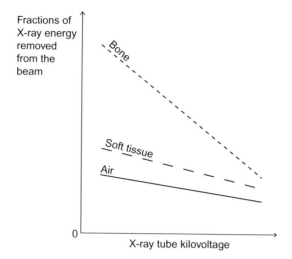

Figure 3.4 Schematic illustration of the effect of kilovoltage changes on image contrast (due to absorption). At lower kV values, larger fractions of X-ray energy are absorbed by skeletal structures than by soft tissue or air, by photoelectric absorption, owing to bone's relatively high effective atomic number. As kV is increased, the fraction of energy absorbed by photoelectric absorption decreases steeply, while fractional reduction due to the Compton process (predominant in soft tissue) reduces only gradually. As a result, the difference between these two, responsible for image contrast, reduces as kV increases: on high kV images, skeletal structures appear less prominent than on equivalent low-kV images. The difference between attenuation in lung tissue and air reduces relatively slightly, as kV is increased, sustaining image contrast when the 'high kV' technique is used for chest radiographs.

radiation intensities within the emergent beam are less varied, and the image contrast that they produce when interacting with the image receptor is reduced (Figure 3.4).

Where tissues or substances within the object attenuate by one process more than the other, either because of *effective atomic number* (photoelectric absorption) or *electron density* (the Compton process), changes in contrast are more selective. The following examples illustrate this point.

Skeletal radiographs

The radiographic distinction between bone and the surrounding soft tissues (fat, muscle) is mainly due to a difference in their effective atomic numbers. For bone, it is approximately 14, while soft tissue has an effective atomic number of approximately 7. To demonstrate this difference as a significant image contrast, a kV should be selected so that it just penetrates the most radiopaque area of interest. When the kV rises above this value, the fraction of energy removed by photoelectric absorption in bone declines steeply, in inverse proportion to the *cubed* value of the kilovoltage. Absorption in soft tissue also reduces, but less markedly, so the difference between these two fractions narrows, and the image has less contrast.

Chest radiographs

Images of healthy lungs show contrast owing to attenuation differences between lung tissue and air. These are due to their electron densities: air has a much lower electron density (i.e. water/hydrogen content) than the lung tissue that surrounds it. (The effective atomic numbers of air and lung tissue are not markedly different, so image contrast is not significantly dependent on photoelectric absorption.) As kV is increased, the contrast between lung tissue and air tends to reduce – but not as steeply as in the case of photoelectric absorption. So, when chest radiography is performed using a '**high kV**' technique, lung field contrast and the image's diagnostic value are sustained. There is an accompanying benefit, resulting from the decline in photoelectric absorption: the fraction of energy absorbed by the overlying ribs reduces significantly; they appear less radiopaque and conceal the lung tissue less than at lower kV values.

The effect of scatter on image contrast

As an absorption process, the Compton process prevents photons from reaching their aligned 'destination' areas of the image receptor. Their absence leaves areas of the image receptor underexposed, in contrast to those where higher transmission has occurred. But because the Compton process makes photons scatter rather than disappear, they retain a potential for affecting the image: if sufficient energy is retained, their random directions inevitably bring some photons to interact with the image receptor. Here, they *cannot* usefully represent features of the object. Unlike the pattern of 'absent' and transmitted photons – which may be regarded a **signal**, scattered photons convey no information; they can be termed **noise**.

The effect of scatter noise is to raise energy absorption across all areas of the image receptor, whether their exposure to the image signal has been relatively high or low. This does not simply make a conventional radiographic (negative) image darker or a positive

Three

screen image brighter. On a radiograph: although scatter darkens low-density areas (where absorption by radiopaque structures has been recorded), other areas where densities are (already) high – i.e. due to photon transmission through radiolucent regions of the object – are less noticeably affected: if exposure has produced full, maximum density, it cannot be increased. So, the effect of scatter is more prominent when superimposed on low (signal) densities; overall, *it reduces image contrast*. An equivalent reduction in contrast is observable in a positive image displayed on a monitor screen: scatter appears to brighten the darker, less exposed areas more than bright areas that have received higher (signal) exposure.

The effect of an increased kilovoltage

When tube kilovoltage is raised, the fraction of energy scattered by the Compton process reduces but, even so, the effects of scatter on image contrast tend to increase. This is because:

■ the scattered photons' energy rises in proportion to the increased energy of the primary photons so they become more penetrating;
■ the angles through which photons are scattered tend to reduce so their travel tends to be more 'forward' – that is, towards the image receptor.

So at higher values of kV, scattered radiation tends to have a more visible effect on the image. When exposure factors are modified by a kV increase, whether manually or when an automatic exposure device (AED) is used, the quantity of radiation reaching the image receptor is adjusted downwards so that the *average* image density (or brightness) stays the same. But these exposure reductions make no distinction between primary and secondary photons and cannot prevent loss of contrast.

The device normally employed to limit the effects of scatter on image contrast is a **grid**, positioned between the object and the image receptor. This distinguishes between scattered photons (removed from the emergent beam) and primary, 'signal' photons (which are allowed to reach the image receptor) on the basis of their direction (see Figure 3.6): primary photons travel along predictable paths from the X-ray tube's target, while scattered photons reach the grid randomly. An alternative, with fewer applications, is a layer of filtering material, e.g. tin or aluminium, placed in front of the image receptor. This absorbs photons according to their energy –

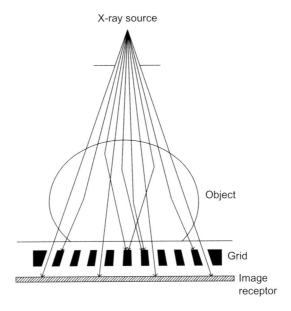

X-ray source

Object

Grid

Image
receptor

Figure 3.6 An anti-scatter grid: 1 – its intended, ideal effect. The transmitted primary photons penetrate the grid's radiolucent channels, and reach the image receptor. Scattered photons deviate from their original alignment with the grid's radiolucent channels, encountering and being absorbed by the radiopaque strips. These effects are enhanced by precise positioning of the grid in relation to the beam: by accurate centring and use of the correct radial distance.

tending to have more effect on the lower-energy scatter than on primary photons.

But a grid and, to a lesser extent, a filter, also absorbs some image-forming, primary photons (see Figure 3.7), so its use must be governed by reference to the *risk versus benefit* relationship.

Kilovoltage selection and radiation protection

The energy involved in production of an X-ray image comprises:

- the fraction attenuated by the object, representing a hazard to the patient, and potentially to other personnel; and
- the fraction transmitted through the object – ideally, entirely absorbed by the image receptor.

The sum of these is constant: so, any factor that increases the fraction of energy transmitted through the object tends also to reduce the radiation hazard to the patient. On this basis, selection of a 'high'

Three

Signal and noise

The difference between these terms, in any context – whether in X-ray image formation, TV or radio reception, or audio reproduction – lies in their contribution to the desired outcome. A signal carries some form of useful information; noise is an accompaniment to the signal that carries no information and, by its effect on the receiver, degrades the clarity of the signal. Maximum clarity is achieved ideally by elimination of noise, but realistically by its reduction, to achieve a high signal-to-noise ratio.

Control of scattered radiation

The harmful effects of scatter, both on the patient and on image contrast, can be minimised by reducing the amount of scatter produced. The volume of tissue irradiated is routinely minimised by primary beam collimation, which limits two of its dimensions, the *width* and *length*. In some further, special circumstances, a so-called 'compression' device may be used that, by *tissue displacement* reduces the volume's *depth*.

Otherwise, the effect of scatter on image contrast is controlled by selectively removing scatter from the emergent beam, before it reaches the image receptor.

Action of an 'anti-scatter' grid

A grid distinguishes between transmitted primary radiation and scatter on the basis of their different directions of travel.

- Primary (information-bearing) photons approach the image receptor along predictable, divergent paths, radiating from the X-ray tube's focal spot.
- Scattered photons (bearing no information) travel towards the image receptor along random paths.

A grid comprises a parallel array of linear, radiolucent channels with opaque walls (formed by very thin strips of lead) aligned to the expected path of the primary beam. Primary photons travel through the radiolucent channels with minimal absorption. Scattered photons, mostly *mis*aligned to the radiolucent channels, tend to be absorbed by the radiopaque walls, and so fail to reach the image receptor.

It is important to note that a grid is not 100% efficient. It cannot prevent all scatter from being transmitted, because the photons' random directions inevitably include some that carry them, unabsorbed, through the radiolucent channels. Inevitably too, the opaque strips intercept and absorb some of the primary radiation photons. So a grid occupies a pivotal position between benefit and risk.

■ Absorption of scatter brings *benefit*, clarifying the image and increasing its diagnostic value.
■ Absorption of information-carrying primary photons enforces an increased *risk* to the patient, because a compensatory increase is required in the amount of radiation, to ensure sufficient reaches the image receptor to form an image.

Fundamentally, a proposed use of a grid has to be justified. Will it significantly raise the diagnostic value of the image? Or, in the circumstances, will the effects of the scatter be insufficient to prevent the image from serving its clinical purpose? (The extra radiation implies a lengthened exposure time that, in some circumstances, may increase the risk of movement unsharpness. Will this prove a greater threat to diagnosis than poor contrast?)

Assuming that it will certainly benefit the patient, accurate use of a well-designed grid must ensure maximising this benefit and minimising the accompanying risk.

The simplest form of a grid has its lead strips arranged to form a linear pattern, parallel in every respect. This is efficient in absorbing scattered radiation (to a variable extent, depending on its dimensions) but is predictably inefficient in transmitting primary photons, particularly towards the lateral margins, because the beam's divergence conflicts with the strictly parallel array of radiolucent channels.

Greater efficiency of primary transmission – reducing the risk, while still presenting a benefit – is achieved by absorbent strips positioned so that their inter-spaces match the rays' divergence. But this improvement imposes a further condition on the grid's use: the distance at which it is used (from the X-ray tube's focal spot) must provide the correct angular beam divergence.

One further problem persists. Positioning of lead strips between the patient and the image receptor implies that their shadows will be superimposed on the (anatomical) image, breaking it up and

Commentary

potentially interfering with its diagnostic value. There are two optional solutions:

(1) precision engineering, to produce *extremely* thin opaque strips, can form a pattern ('lattice') that is virtually invisible;

(2) the use of movement across the grid's lateral axis (at 90° to the strips/inter-spaces) during the exposure, blurs the grid's shadow, so it effectively disappears from the image. This is achievable by mounting the grid within a sprung, oscillating frame, positioned just in front of the image receptor, which is set in motion just before the exposure starts, and continues to oscillate until after the exposure has ended. This device is traditionally known by the name of its inventor, Dr Bucky.

When a grid is used, shouldn't the kV be increased, to compensate for absorbed primary radiation?

The grid's purpose is to enhance contrast, while the effect of an increased kV is a contrast *reduction*, suggesting a possible negation of the benefit. Grid absorption removes a quantity of radiation energy, which is most easily restored by an increase in the *mAs* factor. Where exposures are automated, this will occur naturally. If exposures are set manually, account must be taken of the grid's factor – the value by which the mAs has to be multiplied (compared with a non-grid exposure) to maintain the image's average density/brightness.

Radiosensitive

This term is used, in a relative sense, to describe body tissues and organs that are known to show an increased biological response to the absorption of radiation energy – i.e. a raised risk level.

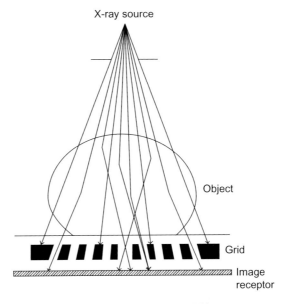

X-ray source

Object

Grid

Image
receptor

Figure 3.7 An anti-scatter grid: 2 – its unavoidable, negative counter-effect. Some *primary* photons are absorbed by the radiopaque strips – requiring a compensatory exposure (mAs) increase, implying a *rise in the radiation hazard* to the patient. Some scattered photons cannot be prevented from penetrating the radiolucent channels and reducing image contrast. These undesired effects can be limited by precise positioning and, where possible, selection of a grid with specifications matching the expected degree to which scatter will affect the image's diagnostic value. *Note:* Bucky movement of a grid has no effect on its primary transmission or its ability to absorb scatter.

kV – i.e. higher than required simply for penetration – appears to be safer than selection of a lower value. This will tend to be true for structures that lie within the primary radiation field. But when the kV is raised, consideration has also to be given to the increased range of the scattered radiation.

The hazards posed by scatter

The effects of scatter on image contrast can be regarded as harmful to the patient, through their potential reduction of the image's diagnostic value. But scattered photons can present a more direct hazard to the patient, and potentially to any person close to the patient who is not fully protected either by distance or by an absorbent barrier.

Three

Hazards for the patient

As kV is increased, scattered photons, though representing a smaller fraction of the beam's energy, have more penetrating potential. So, there will tend to be an increase in the radiation dose to structures adjacent to the volume of tissue irradiated by the primary beam. If some of these are more **radiosensitive** than those within the primary volume, it is possible that raising the kV will increase rather than reduce the radiation hazard to the patient.

Hazards for other personnel

During an exposure, photons are scattered from the irradiated object, forming a radiation hazard within the near vicinity. The concept of a controlled area is an important safety measure. This comprises two parts:

(1) the whole length of the primary beam's path: from the X-ray tube, through the irradiated region of patient's body, until the beam reaches a significantly absorbent barrier (such as a lead screen or a brick/concrete wall); and

(2) an imaginary sphere, centred on and surrounding the patient, within which the intensity of scattered radiation is considered potentially harmful. Like primary radiation, scatter's penetration varies with kV. So, the radius of the sphere increases in proportion to the tube kilovoltage. A radius of 2 metres may provide safety under most conditions, but it is usual for designated controlled areas to be defined by solid, rather than imaginary boundaries.

Radiation protection regulations require all personnel in attendance during an X-ray examination to be outside the controlled area. This normally involves standing behind a fixed protective barrier. If, exceptionally, any persons are allowed to remain within the controlled area – e.g. relatives or friends accompanying an anxious child or supporting an unsteady, elderly patient – they must first receive explanations and safety instructions, give their written consent, and be supplied with appropriate protective garments.

Three

Chapter 4
Formation of a visible image

Introduction

The X-ray beam emerging from an object carries diagnostic information as a pattern of varying intensities: an invisible 'radiation image'. It becomes visible through the action of an image receptor. For over a century, this has been either:

- a photographic film, normally exposed with the aid of intensifying screens, then chemically processed to become a radiograph; or
- a fluoroscopic screen, with electronic amplification and display, presenting a dynamic 'real time' image.

Though still in use, these two types no longer hold a monopoly: increasingly, they are being replaced by systems based on image digitisation and computed image construction.

Some characteristics of an image receptor

Image receptors can be assessed and compared according to many criteria: cost, durability, ease of use, reliability, etc. In this survey, three characteristics will primarily be mentioned, with reference to how each image receptor supports the *benefit versus risk* relationship.

Fluoroscopy / Radiography

X-ray images can be either dynamic (fluoroscopic) or stationary (radiographic) depending on whether there is a need to watch the patient's body in motion or simply record stationary images.

Density / Brightness

The term *density* in its photographic sense describes the extent to which an area of a conventional radiograph has been darkened by exposure. It is measured as the logarithm of the ratio between the light intensities (a) incident on the area and (b) transmitted through it. There is no unit of density; just the logarithmic number. The corresponding feature of a positive image – e.g. displayed on a fluorescent screen – is an area of brightness.

Resolution *versus* speed

Selection of an image receptor tends to involve judgement based on the conflict between resolution and speed: high resolution is almost always associated with reduced speed, while lower resolution may be the cost of increased speed.

Selection must be informed by circumstances:

■ If *movement* is likely to be the cause of image unsharpness, an image receptor's speed is its most important consideration.

■ Also, if radiation protection is particularly important – for example, because the anatomical area being examined contains significantly radiosensitive tissues, or the patient is going to receive a series of exposures, rather than just one – speed will again be a priority.

■ But if radiation protection is *relatively* less significant than the importance (for achieving a diagnosis) of visualising image detail; and *both* immobilisation and beam geometry pose no difficulties, a high resolution is likely to be the preferred option – offering the patient a *Benefit* greater than the *Risk*.

X-ray film construction

Unlike the type of photographic film used in a camera, X-ray film is normally double-sided, with seven layers.

Speed

An image receptor system's speed indicates the efficiency with which it converts radiation energy into a visible image. It depends on two properties:

▪ *X-ray energy absorption* – an ideal image receptor absorbs a high percentage of the emergent beam's energy; and
▪ *conversion of the absorbed energy* – absorption of energy alone doesn't make an image receptor 'fast': the absorbed energy must also be converted efficiently into a form that can produce an image.

The significance of an image receptor's speed depends on whether its purpose is to display **fluoroscopic** or **radiographic** images.

▪ The speed of a fluoroscopic image receptor, exposed to a continuous or pulsed X-ray beam, determines the beam intensity required for forming an image. A fast image receptor requires a relatively low beam intensity, so its high speed is a direct and important factor in protecting the patient.
▪ A high speed brings the same advantage to a radiographic image receptor: the radiation risk to the patient is reduced. But because a radiographic image is formed by a single exposure, the requirement is expressed as a *quantity* of radiation energy, rather than a continuous *rate*. For this reason, high speed brings a further benefit. It is usually possible to deliver the smaller quantity of X-ray energy required by a fast radiographic image receptor in a short(er) time. This reduces the opportunity for movement to occur; so, as well as limiting the radiation hazard to the patient, fast radiographic image receptors reduce the risk of movement unsharpness, and potentially increase an image's diagnostic value.

Contrast

An ideal image receptor is sensitive to every variation of the emergent X-ray beam's intensity and is able to reproduce these as the different image (photographic) **densities** or degrees of **brightness**, depending on how the image is displayed. This important property is fundamental to an image's contrast and invariably to its diagnostic value. An image receptor's contrast characteristics are typically shared between (a) the materials that initially absorb the

Four

- At the centre, there is a clear, plastic *base*, strong and impervious to chemicals.
- Coated onto the base, on both sides, are the film's *emulsions*, which contain extremely small crystals of light-sensitive chemical salts, dispersed within gelatin.
- An adhesive layer, a *substratum*, attaches each emulsion to the base.
- An outer *supercoat* of clear gelatin gives the underlying emulsion some protection against damage when being handled.

Silver halides

Elements within the *halogen* group, significantly iodine, bromine and chlorine, form salts, termed *halides*. Their chemical reaction with silver produces a silver halide. These salts are sensitive to light, and form the basis of most photographic emulsions. Silver bromide is the principal salt in X-ray film but silver iodide is also used.

Latent image

This is the pattern of invisible changes produced within an image receptor, such as a photographic emulsion, by exposure to X-rays or light. It can be detected only when it becomes visible, through the process of development. Exposure ionises the silver halide crystals, making them chemically distinguishable from unexposed crystals. The acquired difference takes the form of a break in the electron barrier surrounding an exposed crystal, opening it to receive further electrons during the process of development. Developing agents convert exposed silver halide crystals into the clustered groups of silver atoms that form the densities (grey through to black) of a radiographic image. Unexposed crystals, their electron barriers still intact, remain protected against action from further (external) electrons – like repelling like – so they stay undeveloped.

Exposure to X-rays produces latent image changes in the photostimulable storage phosphor coated onto a computed radiography imaging plate. These are revealed when the plate is 'read' by laser scanning and the signal has been electronically processed.

emergent X-ray beam, and (b) the photographic or electronic processing that completes the production of a visible image.

Resolution

X-ray image sharpness depends on the beam's geometric characteristics, and a *radiographic* image additionally depends on whether the object has been successfully immobilised throughout the exposure. But these factors concern the pattern of radiation intensities *carried by the emergent X-ray beam* – i.e. at an interim stage, before the image becomes visible. An image receptor's resolution is a measure of the precision with which it preserves the boundaries of each area of intensity within the emergent beam. If it achieves this with point-by-point accuracy, resolution is high and diagnostic information is faithfully recorded. Otherwise, an image receptor that has lower resolution may introduce unsharpness and potentially reduce the image's diagnostic value.

Types of radiographic image receptor

Photographic film

There are differences between X-ray film and the type of film used in a camera but, in both cases, the film emulsions contain microscopically-small crystals of light-sensitive salts, **silver halides**. When exposed to X-rays, visible light or ultraviolet radiation, the crystals absorb energy and undergo invisible changes, together forming a pattern, termed the **latent image**.

Resolution

An emulsion's resolution is determined by the size, shape and distribution of the sensitive silver halide crystals. High resolution is associated with extremely small crystals within a relatively thin emulsion layer. Manufacturers also incorporate additives within emulsions, to enhance resolution.

Speed

Film is thin and easily penetrated so, despite containing elements with moderately high atomic numbers (silver: 47, bromine: 35, iodine: 53) energy absorption efficiency tends to be disappointingly

Four

low. The use of two emulsions doubles a film's ability to absorb X-ray energy but, even so, it is relatively slow when used on its own. For this reason, X-ray film is almost invariably used in combination with intensifying screens (see below). Intra-oral dental radiography is the only common exception to this practice – where use of a cassette presents difficulties.

Contrast

A radiographic image's contrast depends on the film's ability to capture energy from the emergent beam in proportion to each variation in its intensity. The combinations of crystal size and the balance between optional silver halides are important but a radiograph's contrast depends crucially on how the exposed film is developed (Figure 4.1)

Photographic film *with* intensifying screens

Intensifying screens are used for virtually every radiographic examination where the image is recorded on film. The film is tightly sandwiched between two screens and enclosed within a lightproof **cassette** (Figure 4.2).

Speed

The combination of film and intensifying screens forms a very much faster image receptor than a film on its own, because it is much more efficient at absorbing X-ray energy from the emergent beam. So, image formation requires significantly less radiation – with two important benefits:

(1) the biological hazard to the patient is reduced; and
(2) exposure times can be shortened, reducing occurrence of movement and the image unsharpness it can cause.

Like a film emulsion, an intensifying screen's speed increases with crystal size and also with phosphor layer thickness. But the relationship is complicated by the wide range of available screen phosphors – much more varied than the silver halides found in film emulsions. Phosphors are compounds of elements that have relatively high atomic numbers – enhancing their absorption of X-ray energy. Each responds to exposure according to the beam's quality, as well as its intensity, and has its own emission characteristics.

Four

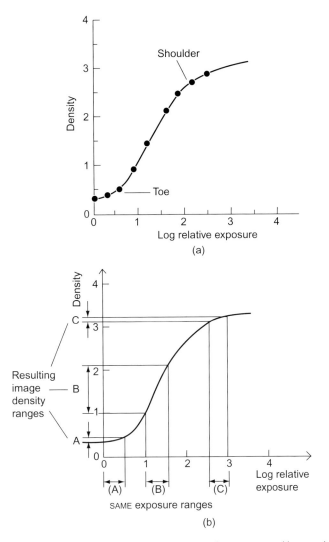

Figure 4.1 Sensitometry – 1: film characteristics. When an X-ray film emulsion is exposed, its absorbed energy forms a latent image. Ideally, absorption should occur *in direct proportion to* exposure energy, *across its whole range*. A graph of this relationship would be a straight line, passing through the origins of both axes. In reality, an emulsion's response is variable. A typical characteristic curve (a) shows four main features of interest. (1) There is an image density, even at zero exposure. This may indicate some non-selective developer action (i.e. conversion to silver of *unexposed* crystals) and it is raised if poorly-stored film has already absorbed energy from other sources before receiving its intended X-ray exposure. (2) Increments of low-value exposure in the curve's 'toe' region are relatively ineffective in building up density: the emulsion is described as having an *inertia* – a reluctance to respond. (3) Between the toe and shoulder, the relationship becomes approximately linear: equal increments of exposure bring proportionate increases in density. The ratio of proportionality, which determines the image's *contrast*, is shown by the curve's gradient; steepness indicates high contrast. (4) In the shoulder region, the gradient reduces: contrast is low, until the density levels off at a maximum value.

(On the horizontal axis, relative exposure values, i.e. they are not measured in absolute units, are plotted logarithmically, to be in keeping with Density, which is naturally a logarithmic value.) Curve (b) illustrates the different image contrasts, A, B, and C, produced by a fixed range of exposure values (typical of the range of intensities found within an emergent beam). This emphasises the importance of avoiding both under- and over-exposure, when exposure factors are selected.

Intensifying screen construction

An intensifying screen is simply composed of four layers – but variations in their composition affect the balance between speed and resolution.

The *phosphor layer* contains very small crystals, suspended within an inert medium. The X-ray energy they absorb is immediately re-emitted as ultra-violet radiation and visible light. The extent to which light spreads out from a phosphor crystal depends on the clarity of the medium in which the phosphor crystals are suspended. A colourless medium allows light to travel relatively far from its origin, tending to reduce the screen's resolution. To limit this effect, manufacturers blend a coloured dye into the suspension medium, shortening the distance the light can travel. But because its action absorbs energy, preventing it from reaching the film, the dye tends to reduce the screen's speed.

This layer is attached to a strong plastic *base* by an adhesive *reflective layer*, which returns light towards the film, originally emitted from the phosphor crystals in the direction of the base. This light would otherwise be wasted – so this layer enhances the screen's speed; but the light's increased spread tends to reduce resolution.

The outer layer, where contact is made with the film, is a thin, protective *supercoat*, to protect the phosphor crystals against moisture and abrasion.

Cassette

A lightproof, protective container, enclosing either a conventional combination of photographic film and a pair of intensifying screens, or a computed radiography imaging plate. Cassettes usually also incorporate identification devices, for marking images with the patient's data. A cassette can reduce the occurrence of image artefacts, provided it is monitored by a rigorous Quality Assurance programme. Otherwise, it can become a collecting point for dust and other matter that can obscure phosphor emissions and become a source of artefacts.

Commentary

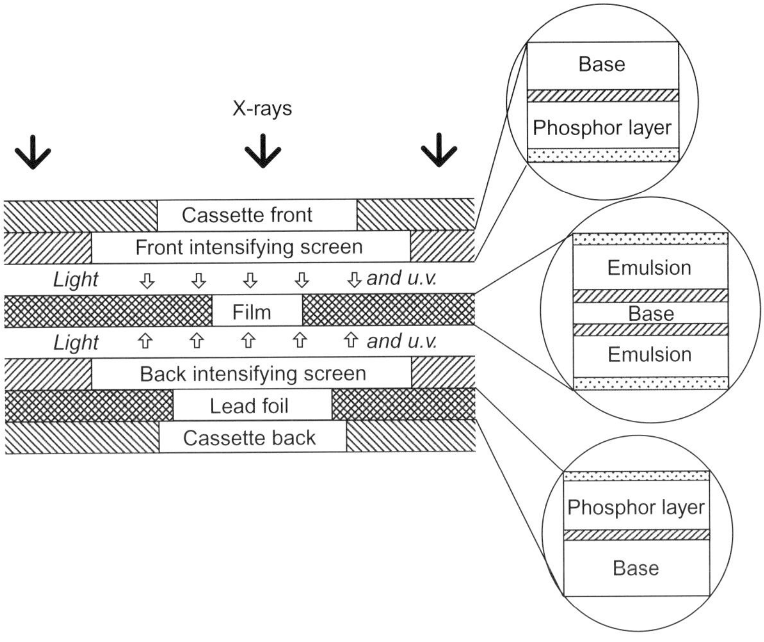

Figure 4.2 Cross-section through a conventional ('analogue') radiographic image receptor. A double-sided X-ray film is normally exposed when held tightly between a pair of intensifying screens, enclosed within a light-proof cassette. After penetrating the cassette front, the X-ray energy (the emergent beam): excites fluorescence of visible light and ultraviolet radiation from the front screen, which is efficiently absorbed by the film emulsion adjacent to it; exposes the film's two emulsions; and excites the back screen, which efficiently exposes its adjacent emulsion. The lead foil and the cassette back (more substantial than the cassette front) form an absorbent radiation barrier.

A film–screen combination's response is maximised if the film emulsion's **spectral sensitivity** is matched to the screens' **spectral emission** (Figure 4.3).

Resolution

An intensifying screen's resolution is influenced by the size, shape and distribution of the crystals and the layer thickness. Again, there is conflict between resolution and speed and, compared with the case of a film emulsion, it tends to be more complex, since an intensifying screen's action involves not only absorption of energy but also energy emission.

Four

Spectral sensitivity

This is the range of visible light wavelengths (colours) to which a photographic emulsion is sensitive, in addition to its sensitivity to X-rays and ultraviolet radiation.

Spectral emission

This is the range of electromagnetic radiations – visible light wavelengths (colours) and ultraviolet radiation – emitted from a phosphor, when stimulated by exposure to X-rays.

Film–screen contact

The resolution of a film–screen combination depends critically on the closeness of contact between the film and the screens. This is achieved initially by a cassette's strength and efficient design: a rigid frame, slight curvature of both the front and back, to eliminate air as the screens close together, and firm clips to lock film and screens tightly together. This efficiency also depends on careful handling of the cassette and periodic checks on the tightness of its hinges and fastening clips. Otherwise, if contact between film and screens is allowed to weaken, radiographs can become affected by irregular, localised areas of image unsharpness. When imposed on the irregularity of an anatomical image, their effect – i.e. the concealment of diagnostic information – can be difficult to recognise. Quality Assurance testing is essential: cassettes must be regularly inspected and tested, using a sheet phantom which has a fine regular pattern, to detect this condition in its early stages, before it can significantly affect patients' radiographs.

Quality assurance

Quality Assurance is a significant and extensive area of professional concern. The modern concept of QA originated in manufacturing industry, with rigorous protocols – production principles, standards and methods – formulated to eliminate imperfections from a factory's products. In the context of a diagnostic imaging service, the 'product' is interpreted as the diagnostic image; but due to its

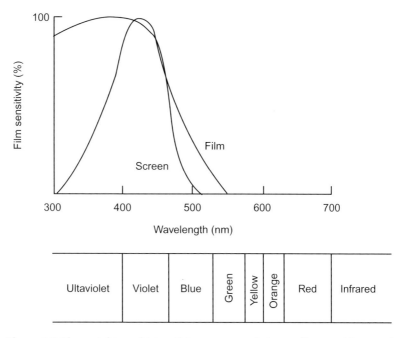

Figure 4.3 The matching of intensifying screen emission to film emulsion sensitivity. Transfer of energy from intensifying screens to film emulsions is most efficient if their emission and sensitivity wavelengths (colours) coincide. Restriction of an X-ray film emulsion's spectral sensitivity – i.e. not extending into the longer-wavelength orange–red regions of the spectrum – allowed these colours to be used for darkroom safelight illumination.

Contrast

Through increasing the X-ray exposure's effect on the film emulsion, intensifying screens also tend to increase image contrast: they enhance the differences between X-ray intensities. In addition, some phosphors have a relatively slow response to low-energy photons, which minimises the effect of scatter; and some low-energy scatter is absorbed by the cassette front and screen base, before it can excite the phosphor layers.

Chemical processing of X-ray film

Exposure of a film, whether to X-rays or light, produces no outwardly visible effects. An exposed film looks just the same as it did before it was exposed: the latent image is invisible. To produce a visible and permanent image, an exposed film must go through a four-stage chemical processing cycle. This comprises development, fixation, washing and drying.

Four

specialised nature, other considerations are essential, notably, the principles of radiation protection. The outcome is a QA programme aiming to benefit every patient alike, typically by ensuring that a patient's imaging investigation is conducted so that it yields the maximum amount of diagnostic information, while exposing the patient to the minimum amount of X-ray energy.

Other aims will be included in an imaging department's protocols, covering, for example, the protection of patients against risks of electrical, mechanical or emotional harm.

It is essential to recognise that a Quality Assurance programme is *preventative*, not reactive. Programme planning involves a series of 'risk assessments', where obstacles to achieving high quality are anticipated and strategies developed to prevent their occurrence. The long-term reward for this approach is a saving of money, time and effort.

Programme implementation requires a professional approach from all staff involved in its delivery: consistent effort, and a belief that quality is important. Threats to success can arise from the fact that some tests and checks yield negative results. When regularly repeated – though actually confirming satisfactory standards – they can appear tedious and unnecessary. To guard against declining effort, staff need encouragement, and the programme needs to be monitored, regularly re-appraised and, if necessary, updated.

Special thought should be given to an important difference between a manufacturing QA programme and one focused primarily on diagnostic imaging quality and radiation protection. The quality of manufactured products (or the lack of it) is usually apparent to the customer – who normally has the right to exercise a choice, to accept or reject. Most healthcare patients are in no position to form a judgement about whether image quality is high, or radiation protection is being fully implemented in accordance with regulations. *Staff have a responsibility of being vigilant on their patients' behalf, to uphold their own high, professional standards.*

White light

This term describes the perceived effect of a mixture of visible wavelengths (colours): a heterogeneous light, presenting a continuous spectrum. In darkroom practice, it indicates the opposite of safelighting – illumination of a specific colour intended, due to its restricted range of wavelengths, to avoid matching a film emulsion's spectral sensitivity.

Development

The latent image becomes visible through selective conversion of *exposed* silver halide into metallic silver. Unexposed silver halide stays unaffected.

Fixation

Removal of undeveloped silver halide from the emulsion makes the image permanent, allowing it to be viewed safely in **white light**.

Washing

When residual processing chemicals have been removed from its emulsions, a radiograph may be archived for a legally specified minimum period without undergoing significant deterioration.

Drying

Removal of surplus water is essential for handling and filing, etc.

Processing chemistry

The special solutions required for both development and fixation are usually purchased in concentrated form, requiring only dilution with water, according to the manufacturer's instructions. Provided that they meet all safety regulations and produce high-quality results, the *exact* chemical formulation of processing solutions is normally of less concern to those who use them, than an effective **Quality Assurance** programme, to monitor consistency. This complements the care taken when the patient is exposed to X-rays.

Developer

Developer reacts with the *exposed* silver halide crystals within a film emulsion; it is said to 'donate' electrons, converting exposed crystals into the minute specks of metallic silver that, massed in groups, give an image its densities: tones of grey or black, depending on the silver's distribution. By reacting with exposed crystals – *not* with the *un*exposed – developer demonstrates its **selectivity** (Figure 4.4). Developers are chemically formulated to have high selectivity, but it falls short of being 100%: if allowed sufficient time, developer

Four

Selectivity

An ability to discriminate between two identified properties; for example:

- A developing agent can distinguish between exposed and unexposed silver halide crystals in a film's emulsion.
- A fixing agent has no effect on the silver within a developed film emulsion but it reacts with the residual silver halide crystals.
- A grid preferentially absorbs scattered X-radiation but allows transmission of the primary photons.

The pH scale

This scale is used to indicate the acidity or alkalinity of a chemical solution. It is derived from a measure of the concentration of hydrogen ions within the solution. The midpoint of the scale, 7, indicates a neutral solution. Values below 7 indicate acidity, with a ten-fold increase for each pH number, in turn: 6, 5, 4, etc. Values rising above 7, up to a maximum of 14, indicate alkalinity – again with a ten-fold increase between each number: 8, 9, 10, etc.

Chemical fog

The term 'fog' is well recognised as meaning an unintentional, overall 'noise' density, cast across a photographic or radiographic image, reducing its contrast. The usual cause is accidental exposure to light or X-rays. But a similar effect can be produced by a developer solution's lack of selectivity, when it reacts with an emulsion's unexposed silver halide crystals, as well as its exposed crystals.

The constituents of developer and fixer solutions

This account is concerned with principles rather than details – many of which, in any case, are undisclosed commercial secrets.

Developer

Developing agents

Although many chemicals are able to 'donate electrons' to silver halide, only a few are selective – able to distinguish between *exposed* and *unexposed* crystals – and so be used as developing agents. Their chemical effect on silver halides is relatively mild, so they tend not to penetrate the electron barrier that still surrounds unexposed crystals.

Developing agents vary in both their speed of reaction and their selectivity. Unfortunately, these properties tend to oppose one another: highly-selective agents act relatively slowly, while the faster-acting agents are less selective. A practical developing solution normally combines two agents with the aim of benefiting from both: (1) a slow, selective agent and (2) one which, although less selective, acts quickly.

Alkali

An alkali is included, formulated to produce a solution with a pH value in the region of 10–11, at which developing agents work most efficiently.

Restrainer ('anti-foggant')

This reinforces the protection given to unexposed silver halide crystals and so helps the developing agents to maintain their selectivity. Its effect on the image is to minimise formation of background chemical fog – hence its helpful alternative (if unattractive) label.

Other chemical compounds included in the developer solution have similar parts to play in the process of fixation. They are described later.

Fixer

Fixing agent

A single chemical serves the purpose of removing unexposed and undeveloped silver halide crystals from a film's emulsions. Though less complex than a developing agent, it may also be regarded as acting selectively: under normal conditions, it has no effect on the developed silver image.

Commentary

Acid

Before it begins removing silver halide from a film's emulsions, the fixer solution has to bring development to a rapid halt. This is achieved by its acidity: it neutralises any alkaline developing solution carried over within the film's emulsions.

Chemicals common to both developer and fixer solutions

The following – in purpose, if not formulation – are found in both developer and fixer solutions: water, anti-oxidant, buffer, hardener, sequestrating agents, wetting agents, and bactericides and fungicides.

Water

This is so common that it sometimes fails to be recognised as a chemical; water is the *solvent*. It softens the gelatin emulsions, allowing dissolved processing chemicals access to the silver halide crystals. As a diluent, it enables solutions to be adjusted to their required concentrations.

Anti-oxidant ('preservative')

Both developing and fixing agents can become oxidised by reacting with air at the solution's surface. The resulting compounds contaminate the solutions and reduce their efficiency. So, anti-oxidant chemicals are included in both solutions, to reduce oxidation rates and convert oxidation products into harmless compounds.

Buffer

Both developer and fixer solutions are formulated for use at specified pH values. Developer requires an alkaline environment (pH typically between 10 and 11), while fixer is an acidic solution (pH typically between 4 and 5). If precautions were not taken, the solutions' pH values would both drift towards neutral (pH 7) because:

- the developer's alkalinity tends to be reduced by hydrogen ions, released into solution as by-products of development; and
- the fixer solution receives recently developed films, bringing with them traces of alkaline developer solution. Unchecked, these would reduce the fixer solution's acidity.

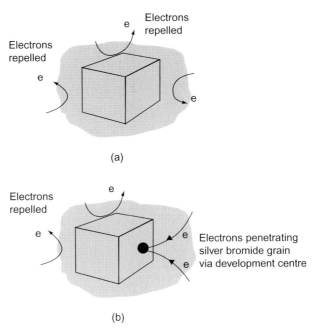

Figure 4.4 Developing agent selectivity. (a) Under ideal conditions, the negative ion barrier surrounding an unexposed silver halide crystal repels the action of a developing agent, leaving the crystal undeveloped. (b) Exposure of a silver halide crystal creates a microscopically small break in the negative ions barrier – a 'development centre' – which permits electron penetration when the emulsion is immersed in developing solution.

action could eventually convert *all* the silver halide into metallic silver. If this were to occur, the result would not be an 'image'; the emulsion would simply form an overall, high density: no contrast, *no information*. So, in practice, development is a process that is necessarily *interrupted* at some point. Calculation of this point is critical: it should be timed to produce maximum image contrast, with optimal distinction between exposed and unexposed areas of the image.

Fixer

When it emerges from development, a radiographic image is vulnerable: its unexposed parts remain sensitive to light and, to some extent, the developer solution retained in the emulsions is still active. So, undeveloped silver halide crystals must quickly be removed from the film's emulsions. This requires chemical action because silver halides are insoluble in water; they cannot simply be removed by washing. This process is termed fixation; the fixer's

Four

So both developing and fixing solutions incorporate chemicals designed to absorb the additional, released ions and maintain the solution's original pH value. These are termed 'buffers'.

The remaining four chemicals are required mainly because of the circumstances in which processing is conducted – in the heated, enclosed environment of a processing machine.

Hardener

Gelatin, the medium within which the emulsion's silver halide crystals are dispersed, freely allows access by the processing chemicals but it suffers from a tendency to become soft when heated. It then becomes susceptible to physical pressure and prone to damage when passing through a processing machine's transport rollers. This weakness is remedied by inclusion in both developing and fixing solutions (and in the emulsion itself) of a hardening agent, to limit how much the gelatin swells, without significantly reducing the solutions' access to the silver halide crystals.

Sequestering agents

Depending on local geology, water can be 'hard' or 'soft'. Hard water has a tendency to deposit a lining of limescale ('fur') inside pipes and vessels. This can cause a processing machine's circulation to seize up. So although machines installed in soft water areas may be expected to operate free from such problems, a sequestering agent – a *water softener* – is included in all chemical concentrates, as a precautionary measure.

Wetting agents

Development and fixation times are so short that it is essential for chemical solutions to act instantly and evenly, across the whole of a film's area. A wetting agent reduces any surface tension that could otherwise allow action to be delayed, producing visible density variations (i.e. artefacts) on a radiograph.

Bactericides and fungicides

The heated, confined environment of a processing machine can encourage growth of bacteria and fungi, particularly where traces of detached gelatin have accumulated. Chemicals to combat this are routinely included in the chemical concentrates.

Washing of radiographs

Thorough washing is essential for radiographs' long-term integrity. Residual traces of fixer and fixation products allowed to remain in film emulsions tend, as time passes, to crystallise and decompose, staining and eventually obliterating the image. This defies the requirement that, as a legal document, a radiographic image must be safely archived, remaining accessible for medical and if required, medicolegal use, for a specified minimum period: up to 10 years, (or for paediatric patients, even longer).

Interlocks

These are devices that link two or more functions, to ensure that they happen safely in a correct order. A common, everyday example is found in household appliances such as microwave ovens or a tumble dryers: the door must be firmly closed before the equipment will operate. A similar arrangement prevents accidents with an auto-processor's machinery.

The rate of energy supply from the processing solutions

Energy supply to the films passing through an autoprocessor depends on the solutions' chemical formulation, temperature, and their state of activity (freshness or exhaustion).

The solutions' original concentrations

Periodically, after thorough cleaning, tanks are filled with fresh chemical solutions, according to the manufacturer's instructions. Care is taken to ensure that the concentrated liquids are correctly diluted and thoroughly mixed, so that both developer and fixer are at their correct levels of activity.

Temperature

Solution temperatures are accurately controlled by a combination of electrical heating, circulation, and feedback monitoring.

Consistency is confirmed by a thermometric display on the auto-processor's control panel.

Replenishment

Maintenance of developer and fixer activity is crucially dependent on correct replenishment. When the first film passes through the tanks, some chemical energy is removed from the solutions so, even if only slightly, their potential for processing further films is reduced. The replenishment system responds to this situation: it is designed to keep chemical activity at its original levels.

■ Replenishment solutions are prepared according to the manufacturer's instructions and stored in reservoirs within or adjacent to the processor, in readiness for use.

■ Arrays of detectors at the film feed aperture measure each inserted film's width and length and send proportionate signals to activate electric pumps that draw replenishment solutions from the reservoirs into the developer and fixer tanks (Figure 4.6). The pumps are calibrated according to an imaging department's average workload. Its profile – whether, for example, there is a high proportion of orthopaedic or thoracic examinations – affects the rates at which developer and fixer are used. The importance of an average setting becomes relevant when equipment failure alters normal workflow patterns; all processors within an imaging department should be set to provide identical results.

Both developer and fixer solutions are circulated continuously through heat exchange units to maintain accurate temperatures, and filters remove debris that could otherwise interfere with the machine's operation and create marks on the images.

Sensitometric monitoring

A programme of regular checks is used to confirm that an auto-processor's replenishment rates are maintaining image density and contrast at the correct levels. The checks are based on processing of sensitometric test films (Figures 4.7 and 4.8). Detected abnormalities can give early warning of malfunction, which can be rectified before it has a significant effect on image quality. The

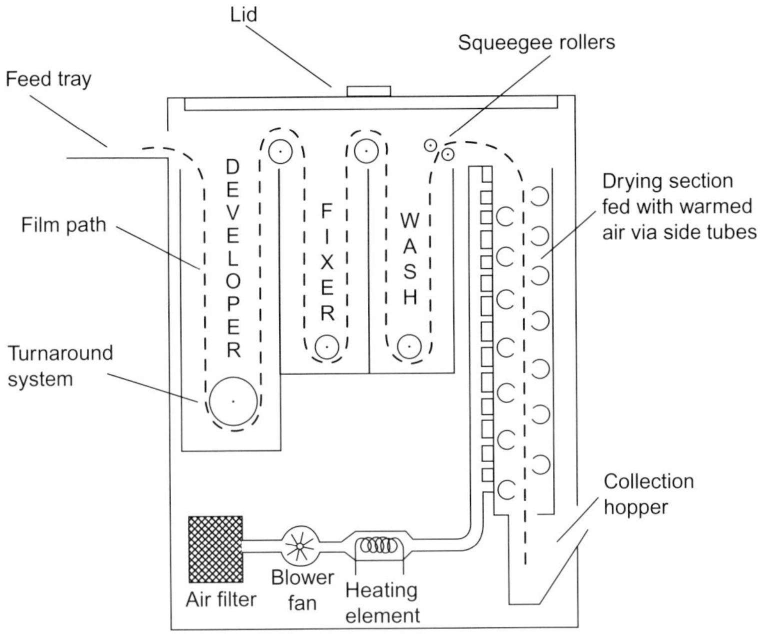

Figure 4.5 Cross-section through a typical X-ray film autoprocessor. Racks of transport rollers carry exposed films through the three liquid 'baths'. Then, squeegee rollers remove some excess moisture from the emulsions, before the radiograph enters the drying section.

purpose is to react with all the silver halide remaining in a film's emulsions, converting it into compounds that are (a) insensitive to light, and (b) water-soluble.

Automatic film processing

A typical automatic processing machine (autoprocessor) is built around a system of transport rollers (Figure 4.5). The rollers collect films from a feed-in tray, then carry them through a line of developer, fixer, and washing water tanks, and finally a drying section.

During processing, films receive energy from the machine, principally from its chemical solutions. The energy acquired by an individual film depends on the time it spends travelling though an autoprocessor and the rates at which energy is supplied. Autoprocessors vary according to their capacities, definable as the maximum number of films that can be processed through a machine per hour. A machine's capacity depends on the sizes of its various sections (e.g. the depth of the tanks) and the length of the film transport path. The speed at which its rollers carry films through the

Four

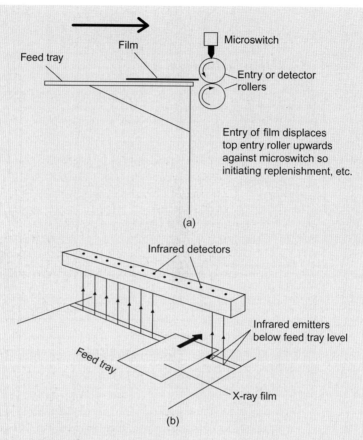

Figure 4.6 Developer and fixer replenishment. Accurate replenishment is essential for maintaining radiographic image density and contrast. Monitoring devices positioned at the processor's feed-in entry point measure every film's length (a) and width (b). Electrical signals from these devices operate pumps that introduce the required amounts of replenisher solutions into the developer and fixer tanks.

preventative nature of this system corresponds with the principles of Quality Assurance.

Prevention of autoprocessing artefacts

Artefacts fall into two general, broad categories: those caused by human error and those caused by machine malfunction, though there is an area of overlap – where machines become faulty as a result of misuse or neglect.

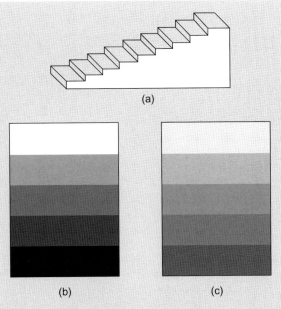

(a)

(b)   (c)

Figure 4.7 Sensitometry – 2: developer activity. A film emulsion's response to exposure cannot be studied until it has become visible through processing. So a characteristic curve (Figure 4.1) essentially *also reveals information about the film's processing* – with attention focused on its development. This is underlined by the fact that sensitometry is an important, central feature of processor QA monitoring.

A simple, long-established method involves exposing a film to a range of discrete energy quantities, produced by X-ray transmission through an aluminium step-wedge (a). The test image is expected to resemble (b), with high contrast, ranging from a minimum density, equated to the wedge's highest step, to a maximum produced by its lowest. Developer deterioration becomes evident when the outcome resembles (c). Overall lack of chemical energy, due to exhaustion, prevents the higher densities from being produced, while loss of selectivity adds to the densities (i.e. creates chemical fog) in higher-step areas, due to development of *unexposed* silver halide crystals.

Despite being simple and inexpensive, X-ray exposure of test films can be unreliable. It has generally been replaced by a commercial equivalent: multi-step test strips produced by finely graded exposure to filtered visible light. Daily processing of these strips enables precise, reliable checks to be performed. (See Figure 4.8.)

Autoprocessors incorporate safety interlocks that prevent incorrect operation (such as feeding in a film too closely after the previous one). Monitoring circuits alert the operator to any accidental malfunction and identify its cause.

Satisfactory machine function depends on cleanliness and attention to regular maintenance, both by local staff and visiting service engineers.

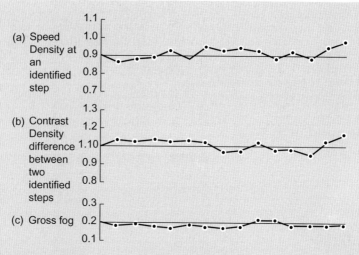

Figure 4.8 A typical QA processing monitor chart. Daily sensitometric checks on developer performance are recorded on a chart, in the expectation that measured characteristics will remain constant – though for every measurement, a narrow *tolerance* is allowed: recorded values that happen to be slightly higher or lower than the standard can be accepted as 'normal'. Typical data include speed, contrast and gross fog. (a) Speed: In this instance, the term is used to indicate how effectively a standard exposure has been converted into a visible form. The density of a nominated step within the test-film's range is measured each time, as a straightforward indicator of the developer's energy supply. If activity, for whatever reason, is high, the 'speed' density will also be high. (b) Contrast: This is measured as the difference between the densities of two nominated steps. It is interpreted as an indicator of the developer's selectivity. (c) Gross fog: The density of a zero-exposed part of the test strip, above or below an established 'norm', reveals the system's performance, with potential implications for image contrast. Simultaneous, accurate measurements of temperature inform interpretation of these results.

Automatic cassette unloading machines have eliminated the handling and darkroom artefacts that formerly affected radiographs.

Autoprocessing: *health and safety* compliance

The working environment is protected against contamination by enclosure of the chemical tanks within the autoprocessor's lightproof, ventilated casing. The solutions' working temperatures are kept relatively low, to minimise emission of fumes. Electrical safety is ensured by the strict regulations enforced whenever electrical and water supplies are used together. Interlocks reinforce physical safety: for

machine tends to be directly proportional to the length of the path: films are transported relatively quickly through a high-capacity machine but more slowly if the path is shorter. So, despite different capacities, autoprocessor cycle times (start to finish) tend to be similar, averaging approximately 60 seconds. An autoprocessor's film transport rate is maintained accurately by a constant-speed electric motor. To complement this accuracy, the rate at which energy is supplied to the films that pass through the machine must also be kept constant.

All processors have design features that guard against the production of artefacts, and they must comply fully with Health and Safety requirements.

Quality assurance monitoring

When applied to processing, the Quality Assurance principle – that all 'products' are of the stated quality, according to defined characteristics – mainly concerns the radiographic images' density and contrast. Both these features of image quality are monitored by visual inspection of patients' radiographs. But it is important to recognise that this form of monitoring is subjective: it is unreliable for systematic analysis of processing quality. Apart from the obvious ethical objection to using patients' images for testing purposes, processor monitoring is an exercise in checking *conversion of the emergent beam into a visible image*. So, exposure must be standardised, free from all risk of misleading variations.

In practice, a series of identically exposed films are processed at regular intervals, from the day when fresh chemicals are first used, onwards. As each periodic check is made, the processed test image is compared objectively with the 'baseline' original. Some tolerance is allowed, to take account of minor, temporary aberrations; but otherwise, the images should confirm that chemical activity remains constant.

Quality Assurance test data can be very comprehensive but an understanding of processing principles is required for their interpretation, enabling early signs of malfunction or deterioration to be recognised.

Four

Computed and digital radiography

Digital imaging has become familiar in the home, particularly through the use of digital cameras, which have displaced the use of photographic film. In the field of diagnostic medical imaging, though digital technology enabled computed tomography, radio-nuclide imaging, ultrasound and magnetic resonance imaging to develop, its application to large-format X-ray imaging lagged behind. A brief look at reasons for the delay forms a useful intro-duction to this survey.

First, there is a significant difference between the comparatively low resolution that satisfies an amateur photographer, and the much higher standard needed for producing high-definition diag-nostic images: the standard set by high quality photographic media had to be matched. Then there is the matter of image size: large radiographic images, especially when coupled with a need for high resolution, require high-performance computers, with large memory capacity and high-resolution display monitors. This equip-ment had to be developed and perfected, and it was important also that it could offer speed, both in the sense of ensuring radiation pro-tection and in its other meaning: quick access to a patient's images, following exposure. Together, these needs demanded a very high computer specification – and so cost (i.e. affordability) came into consideration.

Before digital X-ray imaging could become viable, some clear advantages had to be offered; otherwise, few imaging departments could be persuaded to replace their well-tried, conventional systems with simply an expensive equivalent. These were (and remain):

▥ The ability to access digital images from virtually anywhere, subject to password-protected confidentiality, within the hospital or further afield. So, for example, patients' images could be sent immediately for shared consultation to a remote place, without geographical limitation.

▥ The integration of digital images with other digitised data – typically identification data and reports.

▥ Compact electronic archiving of digitised images to a degree that bears no comparison with the extensive spaces required for bulky, plastic sheet radiographs.

▥ Archive reliability and security, that safeguards digital images against accidental loss.

Despite its cost, the trend for conversion from conventional to digital X-ray imaging continues. At the time of writing, diagnostic imaging departments have the choice between two distinct systems, known as computed radiography (CR) and digital radiography (DR). Both are fully compatible with picture archiving and communication systems (PACS) but the choice of purchase needs to be based on other considerations – for example, what happens to patient care in the event of a system breakdown. Each has its merits and limitations,

Digital radiography

This is the more recent system and is based on 'direct capture' technology. The image receptor is a solid-state thin-film transistor (TFT) matrix, permanently connected ('hard-wired') to a computer, which captures and converts the emergent beam energy directly into an electronic signal that is suitable for handling by a computer system and memory. The imaging process is very fast, requiring no more than 3 seconds from acquisition (or 'capture') to viewing but the equipment tends to be very expensive and its integration into existing X-ray equipment (buckys, couches, etc.) can pose practical problems.

In common with many other new technologies, its increased complexity and capabilities are accompanied by fewer 'moving parts'. So, with a direct capture system, there may be no cassette or image receptor to handle; instead, it is built into the table. Otherwise, there may be a moveable detector for placing into a couch's bucky tray or – for limb radiography, for example – directly in contact with the patient. At the moment, because they need to be hard-wired into a couch or stand, most DR systems are deployed within departmental X-ray rooms. In the event of detector breakdown, although it is theoretically possible to substitute a conventional film/screen cassette or CR plate, it is more probable that the room will be out of action pending the visit of an engineer.

Recent developments mean that DR detectors can be attached to a mobile radiography unit. But the permanent connection of a single size of detector limits the equipment's versatility; it is probably easier to use a cassette. There is also a risk that, away from the relatively protected conditions of an X-ray room, a detector may suffer physical damage and prove very expensive to replace. But it must be added that these may be temporary limitations; future developments could make direct capture radiography a feasible proposition in mobile situations.

Four

Computed radiography

Though indirect and slower, CR is more easily assimilated into an existing imaging department than digital radiography, and it can

example, by preventing the machine from functioning unless its enclosing doors and lids are securely closed. Responsibility to the wider environment is respected by automatic reversion to stand-by conditions during quiet periods when the machine is inactive, to ensure economic use of energy and water. Waste discharges from the machine are filtered and, if necessary, separated out from usual drainage channels. This precaution particularly applies to outlets from the fixer and wash tanks, to prevent release of silver into the water-courses. Despite being a precious metal used for jewellery, silver is a pollutant, as far as environmental conservation is concerned.

Algorithm

This is a set of mathematical formulae that programme a computer used for specific, complex calculations.

Scanning

The process of scanning is employed in many areas of diagnostic imaging. It simply involves a systematic examination (e.g., line-by-line, angle-after-angle) of a relatively large area or volume by a small, precise detector, in circumstances where an instant 'all at once' examination is not feasible. The detector's motion can be electronic, as in a television camera or monitor, or mechanical, as in computed tomography. The data collected during the course of a scan are co-ordinated and combined in the processes of image construction.

Laser

This is an acronym representing Light Amplification by Stimulated Emission of Radiation. Laser beams are used for data detection in a wide range of circumstances – probably most commonly in compact disc players.

Sampling

The process of regular, periodic measurement used to convert an analogue signal into a digital signal. Accuracy of conversion

work out less expensive when installed in a large, multi-roomed department. It requires no changes to the X-ray equipment, so a relatively simple 'overnight' switch can be made from conventional imaging. As far as the X-ray examination itself is concerned, there are few differences between CR image receptors and the conventional use of film and intensifying screens: cassettes are the same sizes and of similar outward appearance. But in CR, the role of a cassette is to act as a lightproof enclosure for a photo-stimulable phosphor plate that stores the energy pattern captured from the emergent beam – paralleling formation of a photographic film's latent image.

After exposure, a cassette is inserted into the identification marker. This permanently links (or 'fuses') the patient's data with the cassette's unique identification data. At this stage also, the digital plate also has an appropriate 'processing' **algorithm** assigned to it, determined by the anatomical area that has been examined. This ensures that the plate will receive correct electronic processing and be optimally displayed.

The cassette is then inserted into a digital acquisition unit – a reader – which extracts the plate and **scans** it with a high-intensity **laser**, at a pre-selected **sampling frequency**. This process converts the stored image into digital data, which are sent to the processing computer. From here, the processed digital signal goes to a work-station, where the image is viewed on a monitor. Meanwhile, still within the data acquisition unit, the phosphor plate is cleared of all previous data by exposure to intense light, and replaced in the cassette which is ejected, ready for re-use. There are similarities here, with the insertion, reloading and ejection of a conventional cassette from a 'multiloader'. But there are similar opportunities, too, for accumulation of dust within the cassette, which can become a cause of imaging artefacts. Special care is taken to eliminate this, within the departmental quality assurance programme.

The preview image

After insertion of a cassette into the data acquisition unit, the time taken for an image to reach the viewing workstation can be a problem, especially in an emergency. To overcome this delay, when the scanning phase has been completed, a small preview image may be available on a monitor built into the data acquisition unit. The preview image is often sufficient for experienced staff to allow workflow to be resumed – for example, for the patient to return to the referring ward or clinic.

Four

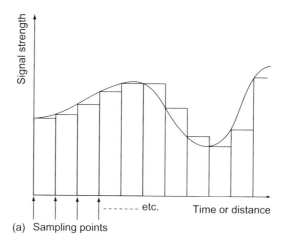

(a) Sampling points

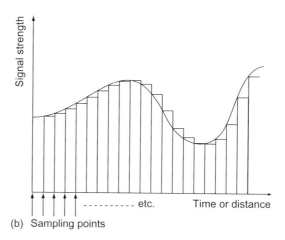

(b) Sampling points

Figure 4.9 Sampling frequency. The reliability of data conversion from analogue into digital, depends critically on the sampling rate. Coarse sampling (a) is unable to follow analogue signal variation as closely as the more frequent sampling (b).

Resolution and speed

To be acceptable as the equivalent of a conventional radiographic image on film, a digital system must offer an equal standard of resolution. Achievement of such a standard can be met despite, as with conventional image receptors, a conflict between speed (which determines the required dose) and resolution. In practice, a compromise may be chosen. The phosphor plates used for general imaging are normally of the same type; there is no equivalent to the choice of fast or high resolution intensifying screens. Instead, the critical feature is the sampling frequency. A high frequency produces high image resolution but reduces the phosphor plate's effective speed. A reduction in the sampling frequency raises the plate's speed but gives a lower resolution image.

Sampling rates are normally preset by the manufacturer and applied by the identification marker to a default value, according to the imaging department's protocol. But a sampling frequency can also be changed. If, in a particular situation, after considering implications for radiation dose and diagnostic image quality, there is a need to alter the sampling frequency from the standard, an override is imposed before the plate is scanned.

The laser reader can cope with the highest resolution of which the imaging plate is capable, so there is no risk of information loss at the scanning stage. Comparisons between conventional (film/intensifying screen) and digital imaging concerning resolution and speed are not straightforward because a digital system uniquely offers the facility of post-processing. This can offset shortcomings in resolution, potentially increasing benefits to the patient, with no added risk. But future availability of different types of plates may be anticipated, extending opportunities even further, for image improvement and dose reduction.

Post-processing

When processed and ready to view, digital images are assessed in a similar way to conventional radiographs: they are checked against standard criteria, according to anatomical coverage, sharpness, lack of distortion, and identification data. But unlike film-based, chemically processed images, which have permanent characteristics, digital images can be electronically manipulated. Manipulation offers the facility of magnifying the image, if this seems likely to increase its diagnostic potential; and particular features can be highlighted by annotation. But two image parameters receive special attention: density and contrast. If they are not exactly as required for a full diagnosis, they can be changed by **windowing**. (Figures 4.10 and 4.11) It is recognised that post-processing takes time that, in a busy imaging department, may be unavailable. So, a department normally has standard protocols for each anatomical area or type of examination, for quick setting of **window level**, masking and the inclusion of alphanumeric data.

Further manipulation may be performed, if required, at the reporting workstation.

If it is departmental practice, some images may be sent directly to the referrer, omitting the reporting stage. A referrer's workstation may have limited manipulation facilities, but the imaging

Four

depends on the sampling frequency: a relatively low sampling rate results in a coarse digital signal that may fail to preserve sudden or subtle variations in the original analogue signal. In a given situation, the rate is set to match the characteristics of the sampled property and the critical needs of the device that receives and processes the digital signal.

Windowing

Digital imaging signals tend to convey a range of image densities (shades, tones) that are too great both for simultaneous display and for the eye to appreciate. Windowing is a process by which this large range can be inspected – through a created electronic 'window' – section by section, so that the whole of the available information can be used.

The window can be moved up or down the range of available densities, to establish a *window level* (or height); and its size (*window width*) can be varied to include the selection of densities that will create an optimum image. These *manipulation* processes can create several images, serving their own diagnostic purposes, from a single set of data, derived from a single exposure. Manipulation of X-ray images can be regarded as a significant aid to radiation protection: there is normally no need for the patient to receive more than a single exposure. Critics have expressed anxiety about the risk of carelessness: they fear that the power of manipulation may be relied on for correction rather than exploration, after the image receptor – and the patient – have been over-exposed.

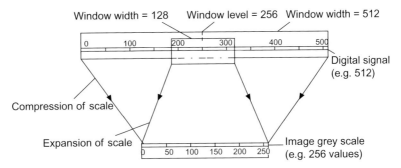

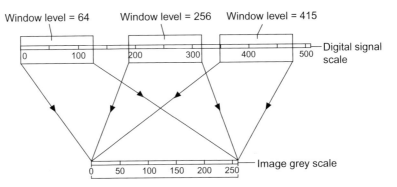

Figure 4.10 Windowing – 1: adjustment of width. The image grey scale comprises 256 digital values. In these two examples, a window width of 512 digital values compresses these onto the image grey scale, for simultaneous viewing, though with some loss of information; with the window width set at 128, there is expansion, so that these selected values fill the grey scale. Both windows are centred on 256.

Figure 4.11 Windowing – 2: adjustment of level. Here, the selected window width is 128. This range of values is shown centred on 64, 256, and 415. In each case, there is expansion onto the 256 image grey scale. These three levels allow closer examination of the range of information contained within the digital signal.

department's manipulated images cannot be affected by actions taken elsewhere.

Archiving

A reported digital image can be archived in more than one place (i.e. copied) with no deterioration of quality. Temporary copies may be kept in hospital wards and clinics, stored on their computers' hard discs, for as long as the images have clinical relevance. But images are permanently stored in the imaging department's main archive: at first, for quick access, on re-writeable magneto-optical

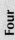

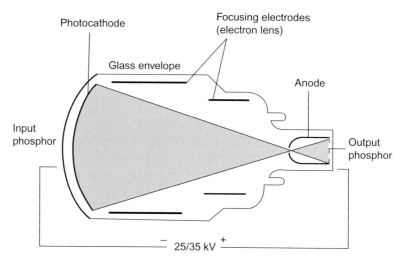

Figure 4.12 Principal features of an X-ray image intensifier tube. The shaded area indicates the path of the electron beam. From its emission at the photocathode, the beam converges to a point at the anode, then diverges to form a small, inverted image on the output phosphor.

discs. Then, after a period of 1–2 years, when clinical relevance has declined, images are typically transferred to more compact but less quickly-accessible digital linear tape.

The introduction of a digital imaging system

An imaging department's installation of a digital imaging system is a major change, especially when it replaces a conventional system that has been in operation for many years. But experience of modern technology suggests that, before too long, updates will be needed, introducing more compact and maybe cheaper equipment, whether to affect a whole system or just one part, such as archiving. Within imaging departments, the change-over to a digital system is likely to occur smoothly, without disruption of services. The various systems' 'friendliness' is an important area for manufacturers' attention. Staff who have experienced this change report opportunities for raising standards of patient care and imaging quality, and enhanced professional satisfaction. Overall, as digital imaging systems become easier to install and afford, conventional radiographic imaging methods are likely to move even more quickly towards obsolescence.

Manufacturers compete also on the excellence of the images their systems produce – perhaps easier to measure than 'friendliness' – from which everyone, not least the patient, can benefit. Guaranteed a high level of image quality, professionals must concentrate their skills even more on the equally important task of optimisation – ensuring that the radiation dose required for every diagnostic image is 'as low as reasonably practicable' (ALARP). A contributory factor is Quality Assurance monitoring of dose levels to identify any drop in detector efficiency – a preventive system giving warning of a need for recalibration or if required, replacement.

There is an impact too upon clinical staff outside the imaging department. Adjustment is needed to cope with technical features – for example, the apparent loss of scale by which a child's thorax on a monitor screen may appear to be the same size as an adult's. There may be a need for training. But until its benefits are recognised, the greatest short-term effect of changeover tends to be psychological, centred on disappearance of the hand-held plastic sheet radiograph and its replacement by an image on a monitor.

Fluoroscopic image receptors

Fluoroscopic images are viewed on a monitor screen. Direct-capture technology is coming into use but conventionally the signal is fed from an image intensifier and a television camera.

Image intensifier plus television

An X-ray image intensifier (Figure 4.12) is a large, cylindrical, evacuated envelope, made of titanium (strong but radiolucent), situated within a protective, shockproofed, steel housing. On all sides except where the input surface receives the emergent X-ray beam, the housing is lined with lead, to minimise X ray leakage. At the back, the housing incorporates a small, circular aperture with a diameter of 3–4 cm, covered with lead glass, through which there is access to the output image. The diameter of the input is normally within the range 30–45 cm. A larger diameter increases the viewable field size but also makes the equipment more bulky. The front of the envelope is convex, so that (to eliminate distortion) there is a constant distance between every point on the input image and its corresponding point on the eventual output image.

Close within the input surface is a layer of fluorescent material that converts the emergent X-ray beam into a visible light image. Intimately applied to the input screen, though electrically insulated from it, is the intensifier's photocathode. This emits electrons where

Four

it is stimulated by light energy, in proportion to the light's intensity. So the emergent X-ray beam's 'image' is converted accurately into an 'electron image'.

At this stage, the electrons emitted from the photocathode (like those produced by an X-ray tube's filament that travel to its anode) are given energy by a kilovoltage (typically 35 kV) applied between the photocathode and the anode. The electrons travel at high speed under the simultaneous influence of electric fields from surrounding electrodes, which focus them to form a converging stream; they reduce to a point at the open centre of the anode. Although attracted by it, the electrons do not actually make contact with the anode; they pass through, then begin to diverge before striking the output phosphor layer. Here, the electrons' energy is converted into visible light, to form the intensified output image. The brightness gain is due to two factors: the energy given to the electrons by the kilovoltage, and the image's size reduction, from the large input, to the much smaller output.

But the image intensifier is a bulky item of equipment and its image quality is dependent on the correct operation of a sequence of stages, some susceptible to malfunction. Instead, the benefits of direct-capture, flat plate technology can modernise fluoroscopic procedures, offering more manoeuvrable equipment, more reliable image quality and reduced radiation doses.

Chapter 5

Computed tomography

Introduction

Conventional radiographs serve a very wide range of diagnostic purposes but there are limits to what they can show. Soft tissue detail and small, low-contrast structures may escape detection, especially where overshadowed by areas of greater radiopacity; and exact spatial relationships between structures (distances and angles) can be difficult to assess. Computed tomography (CT), invented by Sir Godfrey Hounsfield, solves most of these shortcomings: it can reveal parts of the body beyond the scope of conventional X-ray imaging, as detailed single-plane images and three-dimensional reconstructions.

The value of sectional imaging

A tomographic technique (now usually referred to as 'conventional tomography') had been in use, producing images of chosen sections through the body rather than the whole body, for forty years before CT was invented. It involves making an exposure while the X-ray tube travels along a short linear or curving path while an aligned cassette moves at the same time, in the opposite direction. Sectional images are produced due to a principle of relative movement: structures outside the chosen section are eliminated from the image by blurring, simply because their shadows travel faster or more slowly than the moving cassette. This technique is still occasionally performed – for example, during the course of intravenous urography:

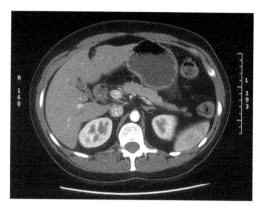

Figure 5.1 A CT image of the abdomen. A 3-mm axial slice through the abdomen at the level of the first lumbar vertebra. A contrast agent has been injected intravenously, and water has been used to distend the stomach, showing its wall. This image (acquisition) has been timed to demonstrate the arterial circulation. (Image by courtesy of the Royal Hallamshire Hospital, Sheffield.)

a relatively thick, posterior section through the upper abdomen can show the renal areas, free from superimposed shadows of (anterior) bowel. But the procedure's simplicity entails a crudeness that limits its use; fine detail is still often unresolved.

CT has retained and developed the value of sectional imaging; it enables small structures to be shown, unobscured by their surroundings, with greatly improved definition (see Figure 5.1) and it has a wide range of image manipulation facilities.

The principles of CT

Multi-angular projection

The two-dimensional limitations of a conventional radiograph are normally addressed by combining the diagnostic information available from two or more projections; *AP and lateral* is a common routine. In some cases, oblique projections are added but, even then, significant features of an object can remain hidden. Computed tomography extends the principle of multiple projections to its logical conclusion: exposures are made while the X-ray tube is driven along a circular path with its beam directed towards the patient's body from all angles, to carry out a 360° survey. Opposite the X-ray tube, across the circle, radiation detectors act as image receptors. At every angle, as the tube encircles the object, an X-ray attenuation profile of the object is recorded. These are analysed by a computer, programmed to calculate the attenuation that has occurred within every part of the chosen body section.

Digital imaging

Conventional radiographs tend to be poor at showing slight differences between soft tissues, because intensifying screens and photographic emulsions have only a limited ability to capture and display minor intensity variations in an emergent X-ray beam. In modern practice, this limitation is addressed by use of digital technology: detectors, not film, measure the emergent beam, producing digitised signals, suitable for computer processing and image construction. But when CT was introduced, radiographic images were recorded exclusively on chemically processed X-ray films. So, central to the success of CT was its pioneering use of digital technology, employing X-ray detectors instead of photographic emulsions, years before it extended into other areas of X-ray imaging.

CT equipment

Over the years since its invention, CT equipment has changed through a sequence of 'generations', each introducing improved electrical, electronic and mechanical designs. These have enabled new techniques to develop, extending CT's diagnostic value. An important factor has been the progressive reduction in exposure times.

Two particular developments of modern CT scanner design and operation are fundamental to their efficiency in producing very accurate, detailed images:

▦ helical scanning movement; and
▦ multislice data collection.

These will be explained later, following an outline survey of the equipment's configuration.

The gantry and couch

The radiolucent couch on which the patient lies is positioned through the centre of a large surrounding frame, termed a gantry

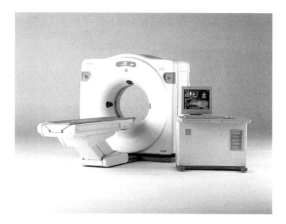

Figure 5.2 CT equipment. The gantry is shown with the couch aligned but not extended into its central aperture. To the right, are the control desk and the computer monitor. (Photograph by courtesy of GE Medical Systems.)

(Figure 5.2). This houses a circular track on which are mounted the X-ray tube and (on the opposite side) X-ray detectors, set out in parallel, linear arrays. The tube and detectors are mutually aligned and freely moveable around the patient, allowing the X-ray beam to be projected through the patient's body from any angle, through a 360° range.

The gantry plane is usually fixed at 90° to the couch, with the X-ray beam passing along normal transverse planes through the recumbent patient; but it can be tilted cranially or caudally (towards the patient's head or feet) through angles of up to 30°. Gantry angulation is useful when examining an anatomical structure that lies obliquely in relation to the body's transverse plane – principally for radiation protection purposes, to shield radiosensitive structures against unnecessary exposure. For example, when scanning the brain, angulation can reduce irradiation of the eye lenses.

The couch is electrically driven, with a full range of travel, long enough to allow any region of the patient's body to be brought into alignment with the X-ray beam, as it passes from the tube across to the detectors. When multiple areas have to be examined, this range allows repositioning to be achieved simply by movement of the couch – a particular benefit for trauma patients.

Production and collimation of the X-ray beam

CT X-ray tubes are specialised and very powerful, capable of sustaining a high-intensity X-ray output and coping safely with the

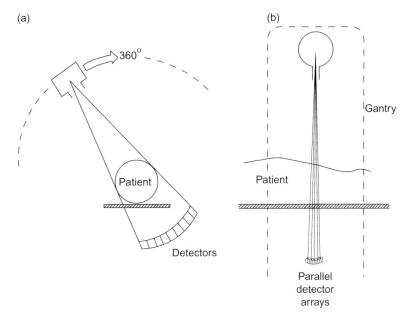

Figure 5.3 CT Beam collimation and centring. Simplified diagram to show the flat, 'fan' beam of X-rays, centred to the curved arrays of detectors, shown from two aspects: (a) along the couch axis; (b) along the plane of the X-ray beam.

accompanying high rate of heat production. Anode discs have a large diameter, typically 20 cm, and a thick, graphite backing that forms a 'heat sink', giving them a very high thermal capacity. Cooling may be enhanced by a circulation of oil, pumped through the tube housing via an external heat-exchange unit. Focal spot sizes normally lie in the range 0.5–1.6 mm². CT generators produce a high-frequency, pulsed, constant potential supply, normally between 80 kV and 140 kV.

Unlike conventional radiography, where the field's width and length are adjusted to cover a whole anatomical region, a CT tube's output beam is tightly collimated by a very narrow, slit aperture to form a flat 'fan'. The narrowness of the beam matches the width of the detector arrays, and its angular spread precisely covers their length (Figure 5.3). Just as when used for conventional radiography, X-ray beam collimation minimises the patient's radiation dose and, by limiting scatter, sustains image contrast.

X-ray detectors

In common with all image receptors, CT radiation detectors ideally have:

- high detection efficiency, absorbing all the emergent X-ray beam's energy to which they're exposed;
- high conversion efficiency, enabling all the detected energy to contribute to image formation;
- a wide dynamic range, so that all X-ray intensities, from weakest to strongest, are converted into proportional output signals.

The detectors are ceramic scintillators, which respond to X-ray exposure by emitting pulses of visible light in proportion to the absorbed energy. The light is converted into electrical signals by photodiodes, coupled to the scintillators, forming compact, efficient units. A feature of modern detectors is their miniaturised size, allowing them to be closely grouped, to enhance the images' spatial resolution.

The CT imaging procedure

Production of a preliminary radiograph

Before beginning the series of CT slice images, it is usual, though not essential, to scan the patient by driving the couch through the fan X-ray beam while *the tube and detectors are stationary*. The outcome resembles a digital radiograph, free from the longitudinal magnification seen on a conventional radiograph. This pilot image, commonly termed a *topogram*, enables accurate plans to be made for the cross-sectional slice series, so that it includes all the relevant anatomical areas but avoids unnecessary, excessive exposure.

The CT slice images

During an exposure, the X-ray tube and detector arrays rotate around the patient. X-ray intensity (attenuation) measurements are made by the detectors, as rotation occurs, effectively dividing the exposed body section into a 'criss-cross' matrix of separate, very small tissue volumes, termed *voxels* (short for 'volume elements') – see Figure 5.4.

Signals from the photodiodes are fed via an analogue-to-digital converter to a computer, programmed with complex, equation-solving, algorithms. These calculate the X-ray attenuation that has occurred within each voxel – effectively, its relative radiopacity or radiolucency. The voxels' attenuation measurements are converted into proportionate grey-scale tones and displayed on the

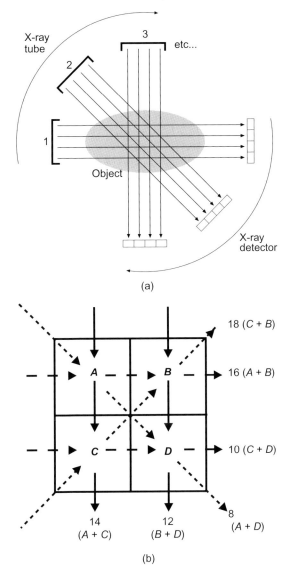

(a)

(b)

Figure 5.4 Multi-angular projection: creation of a matrix and measurement of values for individual voxels. These diagrams illustrate two principles of the CT process: (a) The circulating X-ray tube projects a beam through the body towards an array of detectors, from numerous different angles. This creates a matrix of voxels within each X-rayed slice. (b) Detector readings are fed to the CT computer, which calculates individual attenuation values for each separate voxel.

Try calculating the values for A, B, C and D, in this simple 2×2 matrix. Detector measurements are shown for simplified horizontal, vertical and diagonal projections.

$B + A = 16$ $B + C = 18$ $\therefore$ $C = A + 2$

But $A + C = 14$ $\therefore$ $\underline{A = 6}$ and $\underline{C = 8}$

$A + D = 8$ $A = 6$ $\therefore$ $\underline{D = 2}$

$B + C = 18$ $C = 8$ $\therefore$ $\underline{B = 10}$

computer's monitor screen, each in its correct position within a matrix of pixels (short for 'picture elements') that together form an image of the exposed section. Typically, an image is composed of approximately 260 000 pixels, arrayed in a 512 × 512 matrix.

It should be noted that, while voxels are three-dimensional, the pixels forming the grey-scale display of their attenuation characteristics are only two-dimensional. Every pixel has a value assigned to it: a *CT* or *Hounsfield number* derived from the attenuation coefficient of the substance represented by the pixel. Being in a digital format, CT images can be manipulated and enhanced by windowing, for full access to the diagnostic information they have to offer.

Features of helical multislice CT scanning

Modern CT scanners differ from earlier equipment in many significant respects. A full comparison would satisfy little more than historical interest but there is value in identifying and explaining some of the key points.

'Volume' data acquisition

Early equipment could only explore body volumes through a series of parallel slice images, each produced by a separate exposure. This was a slow procedure and continuity or registration between adjacent slices was unreliable, particularly if arrested respiration was required.

During a helical CT scan:

■ the X-ray tube encircles the patient continuously, while
■ simultaneously, the table is driven at fixed speed through the gantry's aperture.

The combined effect of these movements is that the X-ray beam traces a helix (a spiral path) through the patient's body, generating data about an entire cylindrical volume, from which images can be constructed, as required (Figure 5.5).

Detector size reduction and multiple arrays

The single detector arrays originally installed on CT scanners enforced slow rates of data collection. In view of the need for immobilisation, this proved to be an obstacle to producing high quality

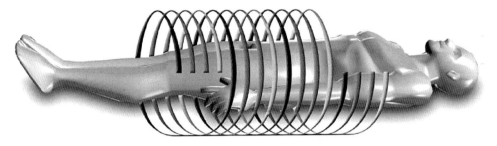

Figure 5.5 The principle of helical multislice CT. As the tube/detector gantry rotates and the couch advances, spiral traces (four shown in this simplified diagram) are formed, generating imaging data about the body volume. (Picture by courtesy of GE Medical Systems.)

images: blurring and artefacts occurred, particularly when patients were too ill to co-operate.

Modern, miniaturised detectors have enabled arrays to be narrowed to as little as a half a millimetre in width, allowing scanners to incorporate multiple, parallel arrays, up to 64. These simultaneously record several slices, speeding up data collection rates and shortening exposure times. Quick, efficient body volume imaging is now possible: the whole chest, abdomen and pelvis can be scanned during one short breath-hold.

Image definition and contrast agent enhancement

Faster imaging techniques and overall improved efficiency have refined the use of contrast agents: following a single injection, both arterial and venous phases of a circulation may be demonstrated across a large body volume, demonstrating small vessels and the structures to which they are related.

Slice width selection

The width of the X-ray beam 'fan' can be controlled, to allow coverage of any required number of the parallel arrays. When used at a wide setting, compensatory adjustment of the detector readings is available to address the problem that, despite the arrays' narrowness, the beam's outer rays pass slightly obliquely through the slice, potentially distorting voxel shape.

Data acquired simultaneously by adjacent arrays can be interpreted individually or electronically combined, to vary slice thickness. For example, sub-millimetre slices through a chest will show fine lung detail. Combined to form a 5-mm slice, they will show improved soft-tissue detail.

Computer capacity and speed

The high-speed data acquisition and processing implied by helical multislicing has become feasible only through the development of computers with large capacity and high-speed operation.

Image processing

Window width and level

When an image's pixels CT numbers are translated into a grey scale image and displayed on the computer monitor, the eye can distinguish fewer shades of grey than the range of attenuation values acquired by the detectors. So, to address this imbalance (which also arises during digital and computed radiography) images may be routinely manipulated to obtain all the information contained within the collected data. Two basic manipulation techniques are adjustment of *window width* and *window level*.

- *Window width* is the range of CT numbers chosen to form an image. Reduction of the window width decreases the range of the grey scale, so that the contrast between relatively similar tissue densities is increased. When imaging the brain, a reduction enables white matter to be differentiated from grey matter. Using the same data, a window width increase enables bone detail to be visualised.
- *Window level* is the centre of the chosen range.

By adjustments to both the window width and level of a single set of data acquired by scanning the thorax, clear demonstration can be obtained of the ribs or the air-filled lung tissue or the mediastinal soft tissue (Figure 5.6).

Reformatting

When a CT examination is carried out, the gantry plane is normally vertical, so, with the patient lying on the couch, transverse sectional images are produced. If other planes (coronal, sagittal, oblique) are needed, it is usual to construct them by reformatting, from the volume data already acquired – i.e. without having to re-expose the patient. They have the same high quality as original transverse images: small, tortuous vessels and fine bony structures can be viewed in multiple planes and as three-dimensional models.

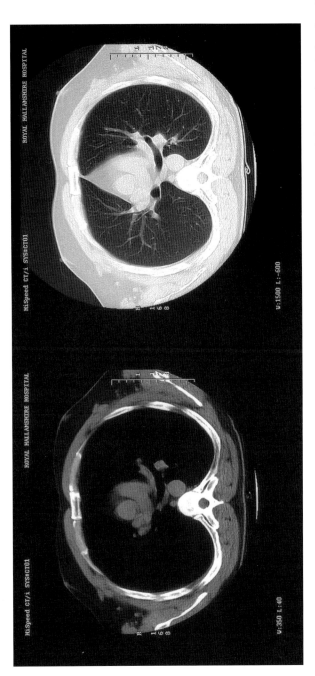

Figure 5.6 The diagnostic value of windowing. By adjustment of window level and width, these two CT images of a section through the chest have been derived from a single set of data – i.e. a single exposure of the patient. (a) A level of 40 and a width of 350 show soft tissue structures (thoracic wall and in the mediastinum). (b) A level of 600 and a width of 1500 show lung detail. (Image by courtesy of the Royal Hallamshire Hospital, Sheffield.)

Storage and archiving

After manipulation and reporting, images can be transmitted to remote viewing stations in clinics and wards, via electronic communication systems. Image data are then archived.

Image quality

CT image quality can be assessed according to five criteria: spatial resolution, contrast resolution, accuracy, noise and artifacts.

Spatial resolution

This term indicates the extent to which small, high-contrast structures situated close together within the object can be identified as being separate structures. As in conventional radiographic imaging, the geometry of the system (focal spot size, focus–object and object–detector distances) exerts an influence. But spatial resolution is essentially affected by the size of the voxels. So, factors governing the voxels' dimensions are relevant: the size of individual detectors, the collimated narrowness of the X-ray beam, and the number of angles at which the circulating tube is energised.

Spatial resolution is also dependent on the object remaining motionless during data acquisition – a further area in which the short exposure times made possible by helical multislicing offers advantages.

Contrast resolution

This term refers to differentiation between structures that have small differences in attenuation. Some of the factors that influence the contrast of conventional radiographs are also relevant to CT imaging: tube kilovoltage determines the relative attenuation occurring within the different tissues, and primary beam collimation controls scatter production. To supplement this action (though not to protect the patient) collimation of the emergent beam can be effective: thin lead barriers (septa) positioned around individual detectors, at their shared boundaries, act in a manner similar to an anti-scatter grid.

The dynamic range and sensitivity of the detectors must be sufficient to enable them to register small differences in X-ray attenuation. Further computer enhancement is possible, using an algorithm designed for this purpose.

Accuracy

Accuracy depends both on how precisely a CT image reproduces its objects' spatial positions and how consistently it records their attenuation characteristics. This is critically assessed by measuring how closely objects that produce uniform attenuation are displayed with the same CT numbers.

The accuracy of the detectors' measurement of attenuation within the voxels is enhanced by their location within curved arrays, equidistant from the X-ray source; but it is potentially reduced by the *beam hardening effect*. Low-energy photons are selectively removed when a heterogeneous X-ray beam penetrates a partially absorbent barrier. This 'hardens' (i.e. it raises the quality of) the beam – an effect deliberately employed for protection purposes, when an X-ray beam is filtered (e.g. by aluminium). But it also tends to occur when the beam passes through any object that is being X-rayed, often most significantly, owing to its contours, through its centre. For a single-exposure radiograph, the phenomenon is hardly relevant but for repeated, multi-angle CT exposures, it can have a detectable effect on measured CT numbers (e.g. when examining the brain in the posterior cranial fossa) unless eliminated by electronic compensation.

Another potential influence is the *partial volume effect*. CT numbers assigned to voxels are averages; so, if a voxel happens to contain a boundary between two tissues differing in their radiopacity, the difference will tend to be smoothed (averaged) out. A reduction in voxel size increases the accuracy of CT numbers, so there is a positive correlation between improved spatial resolution and accuracy.

Noise

Noise, the random energy that accompanies *but is unrelated to* a signal, can cause unreliable variations in CT numbers, and is particularly noticeable within areas where attenuation is uniform. The type of algorithm used for image construction may affect the prominence of noise, and there are three other potential influences: pixel size, slice thickness, and exposure magnitude. Control of these factors is not straightforward; negative and positive must be balanced against each other. The effects of noise are reduced:

■ if pixel size and slice thickness are increased – both these changes decrease spatial resolution;
■ if the exposure is increased – but this raises the dose to the patient.

These examples illustrate the conflict often involved in selecting imaging parameters, and underline the need for experienced and specially qualified staff.

Artefacts

Artefacts are features appearing within an image by accident, seemingly representing structures that are not actually parts of the object. Helical multislice images suffer much less from artefacts than earlier technologies, through reductions in voxel size, slice thickness and exposure time.

Preventative QA programmes normally eliminate the characteristic artefacts associated with equipment malfunction.

Quality Assurance

As with all imaging modalities, a rigorous QA programme is essential. Its value lies in early identification of anomalies and trends, which can then be eliminated before image quality begins to deteriorate or radiation dose unnecessarily increases. Aware of their responsibilities, equipment manufacturers advise sequences of test procedures appropriate to their particular equipment, and recommend frequencies at which they should be performed. Most involve scanning a special CT phantom (typically a water-filled plastic cylinder, containing various test patterns) supplied by the manufacturer. The routine test procedure is relatively quick: often, a single scan is sufficient to enable the operator to measure the various parameters.

Tests are performed and record-keeping starts with the first post-installation check, when the equipment is new. This is when baseline criteria are established, against which all future results are measured. By following these procedures, gradual deterioration is detected early, before it begins to have a significant effect on either image quality or radiation dose. Ideally, tests confirm the equipment's consistency. It is recommended that daily calibrations are carried out and weekly checks are made on CT numbers, noise and uniformity.

- ▦ *High-contrast* resolution is tested by using a pattern containing rows of holes of varying sizes. A record is made of the smallest row in which the holes can be identified as being separate.
- ▦ *Low-contrast* resolution is measured by using a pattern composed of discs of varying density; again, the test involves identifying critical separate elements within the pattern.

Equipment performance is supported by regular servicing; intervals vary with the equipment's age and its workload. External checks on accuracy, image quality and radiation safety are performed annually by specialist technicians, and routinely repeated after any major repairs or modifications, such as the installation of a new X-ray tube.

Regular quality assurance is mandatory to comply with ionising radiation regulations but the programme – particularly if it is quick and easy to perform – ensures continuity of service (reduction of equipment 'downtime') as well as optimal image quality and safe operation.

Patient care and management

Patient care is achieved across a broad spectrum of factors. The time-saving features of helical multislicing, though primarily associated with image quality, also offer the chance to shorten waiting times.

Radiation protection and image quality

Some selected actions can reduce radiation dose to the patient or enhance image quality, without negative consequences. For example, X-ray beam collimation is wholly positive in its effect; and regular equipment servicing, supported by a rigorous QA programme, enhances both radiation protection and image quality improvement without compromise.

But in CT, as in other areas of X-ray imaging, some strategies intended either to reduce radiation dose to the patient or to enhance image quality, can have a contradictory effect. For example, a reduction in the amount of X-ray energy used for imaging (to protect the patient) may negatively increase image noise, causing deterioration of image quality. These possibilities underline the critical need for staff to have full knowledge of their equipment; skilled evaluation and judgement, and their ability to balance all factors, can produce optimum diagnostic images with the minimum amount of radiation dose.

Operator skill is required in all imaging modalities but there is a particularly important reason for emphasising this matter in relation to CT. Continuous technical development has probably brought CT to a point at which *a gap is appearing between the high-quality images that can be achieved and the standard that is actually required for diagnosis.*

Computed tomography's remarkable contribution to medical practice is a tribute to its inventor. But it must not be allowed to conceal the fact that CT images are derived from exposure to X-radiation, with all its inherent biological hazards, and that CT is regarded as a high-dose procedure. In the UK alone, there is a huge (maybe ten-fold) disparity between the nationwide use of CT expressed as a percentage of all diagnostic X-ray examinations, and CT's percentage contribution to the national annual collective radiation dose.

The accessibility of CT, enhanced by the operational speed of modern equipment and the quality of its images must not be allowed to deflect attention away from the high doses involved. Referring clinicians may need to be reminded that this imaging modality is governed by the same strict criterion that applies to all X-ray techniques: *benefits must outweigh risks.* CT should never be used if equally effective and less harmful alternatives are available.

Future developments

Increased data acquisition speeds and higher image resolution have extended the scope and accessibility of CT. Visualisation of narrow tortuous vessels has made CT angiography more common, increasing the diagnosis of vascular abnormalities – e.g. in the cerebral and cardiac circulations.

Reduction in respiration and peristalsis movement artefacts, and the high quality of reformatted images have led to the development of virtual endoscopy, which opens the possibility that CT will be used more widely for colonic and lung screening. CT will also develop as a fast and effective tool in the assessment of major trauma, through demonstrating damage to soft tissue and bone in multiple areas of the body.

Chapter 6

Radionuclide imaging

Introduction

Nuclear medicine has two branches:

(1) the treatment of disease by means of radioactivity; and
(2) diagnostic procedures, using radioactive materials.

Procedures can involve either analysis of samples (generally called *in vitro* tests – literally, 'in glass') or examination of the living body ('*in vivo*'). This chapter is concerned with *in vivo* imaging of the body, using a gamma camera to detect gamma-emitting radionuclides, introduced into the body, most commonly by injection of a radiopharmaceutical.

Nuclides are atoms specified by their atomic numbers and mass numbers – i.e. by the numbers of protons and neutrons within their nuclei. *Radionuclides* are unstable nuclides in the course of becoming stable, adjusting their nuclear components by conversion or emission of particles and radiant energy. These processes are termed *radioactive decay*.

Radionuclide imaging procedures do not duplicate the information obtainable from X-ray imaging; they have their own, separate diagnostic value, due to two important facts.

(1) Radionuclide images of an organ or other body structure show its *function*: they primarily demonstrate physiology rather than anatomy (see Figure 6.1). So, unlike X-ray imaging, which tends to be used for examining *areas* of the body, RNI demonstrates specific *organs* or body *systems*.

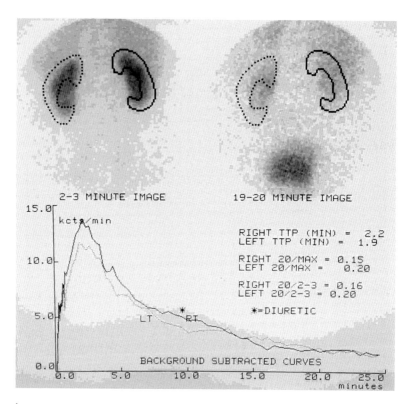

Figure 6.1 A renogram. This RNI examination of the renal tract yields graphical information about kidney function, and images that, in this case, show both kidneys functioning within normal limits. The early concentration of radiopharmaceutical in the kidneys is followed by drainage into the urinary bladder. (By courtesy of King's Mill Hospital, Mansfield.)

(2)   Many diseases can be diagnosed through disordered function of the affected organs or systems *much earlier* than when shape and physical appearance have become affected. In other words, RNI can reveal early pathological changes, ahead of imaging methods that demonstrate disease through structural change.

There are practically no similarities between X-ray and radionuclide imaging: the techniques are fundamentally different. But X-rays and gamma rays are both ionising radiations, so radiography and RNI are together governed by an important, common principle, *optimisation* of exposure: obtaining maximum diagnostic information while exposing the patient to the minimum amount of radiation.

Production of gamma radiation

A radionuclide has to be selected to suit the specific organ or body system being investigated. This involves three main considerations: type of emission, half-life and photon energy.

Types of emission

Many elements occur in radioactive forms but are unsuitable for use in RNI because, as well as gamma rays, they also emit alpha and beta particles.

▪ *Alpha decay* occurs when, in a effort to become stable, the radionuclide emits *alpha particles* from its atoms, each comprising two protons and two neutrons (i.e. a helium nucleus). Being relatively large and positively-charged, alpha particles do not travel very far in tissue, and so they deliver a high local radiation dose to body tissues. The short distance prevents alpha particles from being detected by an imaging device outside the body.

▪ When *beta decay* occurs, a negatively-charged particle equivalent to an electron, is emitted from the nucleus. Beta particles are also soon absorbed by surrounding tissue – again, contributing to the dose received by the patient but not to formation of the image.

▪ *Gamma rays* are a form of electromagnetic radiation: high-energy photons that can pass easily through tissue and be detected by equipment outside the body. So, for image formation, *radionuclides must be gamma ray emitters*, while for the patient's safety, they *must not emit alpha or beta particles*. Exclusion of alpha and beta emission serves a similar purpose to the filtration of an X-ray beam: removal of low-energy photons that are incapable of contributing to image formation.

Half-lives

Physical half-life

Because it is an emission from a radionuclide, not the product of energy conversion within electrical apparatus, gamma radiation cannot be used in the instant 'on' / 'off' manner of an X-ray exposure. The radioactive processes that produce gamma radiation

Six

proceed at predetermined rates; they cannot be stopped, slowed down or speeded up. Radioactivity reduces according to the natural physical law of exponential decay: a fixed percentage reduction occurs over a given period of time. This means that future levels of radioactivity can be predicted accurately. While the time taken for a quantity of radioactivity to reduce to any given percentage can be calculated, it is standard practice (and convenient for comparing radionuclides) to identify the time taken for radioactivity to fall to specifically 50% of its original value. This is termed its *physical half-life*; it is a property unique to each radionuclide.

Biological half-life

Some radionuclides can be used in their original forms, such as when a radioactive gas is used to measure respiratory function. But much more commonly, radionuclides are combined with – they are said to 'label' – non-radioactive chemicals, termed 'carriers', to form *radiopharmaceuticals*. These are formulated for introduction into the patient's body, to be taken up – e.g. by diffusion or by metabolic activity – and concentrated within specific cells and tissues.

Radiation exposure hazards to the patient are related to the radionuclide's physical half-life but also to the time that the radiopharmaceutical remains within the patient's body. The concept of *biological half-life* indicates how quickly a radiopharmaceutical is excreted or otherwise removed from the body; specifically, it is the time taken after its introduction for the amount left in the body to reduce to half its original value.

Effective half-life

The overall radiation dose to the patient is affected by *both* the physical half-life (indicating the radionuclide's rate of decay) and the biological half-life (which depends on the rate of the radiopharmaceutical's removal from the body). These combine into a property used in dosimetry calculations, termed the *effective half-life* – meaning the time taken for the amount of radioactivity left in a patient's body to reduce to half its original value.

Doses are carefully calculated to ensure an accurate and appropriate effective half-life. Otherwise, if it is too short, radioactive emissions may decay to an undetectably low intensity before imaging is completed; and if it is too long, the patient (and possibly other people) will continue receiving a radiation dose for an unjustified period after the examination has been completed.

Photon energies

Gamma radiation and characteristic X-ray photon energies share a similarity: they have fixed values and form line spectra, measured using the same unit – the kiloelectron volt. Some radionuclides emit multiple photon energies, as several line spectra (*not* a continuous spectrum) – requiring the imaging equipment to have multiple detector settings. Others, being single energy emitters, are easier to detect.

The primary purpose underlying selection of an X-ray tube kilovoltage is penetration of the object: ensuring that the emergent beam contains sufficiently energy to form an image. Penetration is also the purpose of gamma radiation energy selection, but in this case the radiation's path only crosses part of the width (or other dimension) of the patient's body. During the imaging process, gamma radiation originates within the organ under investigation, so its required distance of travel may be as close as the nearest skin surface.

Gamma photon energies suitable for RNI imaging – able to reach the radiation detector/image receptor outside the body (normally a gamma camera) – lie between 70 keV and 350 keV. Below this range, photon detection would be inefficient: imaging signals would be weak and unreliable. Above this range, photons would tend to over-penetrate the detectors; energy would be wasted instead of being used efficiently, and the photons' ionising effect on the body could spread to affect an unjustifiably large volume.

Radiopharmaceuticals

Radiopharmaceuticals are formulated under very strict conditions of purity (non-toxicity) and imaging efficiency, and administered with accuracy. These precautions ensure:

▧ rapid uptake and concentration within the specified cells and tissues, to provide a reliable indication of normal or abnormal function;

▧ safe distribution and uptake in (or close to) critical organs such as the urinary bladder wall;

▧ efficient removal from the body over a period comparable to the expected time of the imaging procedure;

▧ a period of activity matching the length of time taken to complete the intended imaging programme – fulfilling the requirement to limit the patient's exposure to the minimum amount of radiation.

Image formation

These procedures are described according to the most common clinical practice: the use of a gamma camera.

After administration of a radiopharmaceutical, provided that the organ under investigation is functioning, images can be obtained that show:

▓ where the radiopharmaceutical has been collected or concentrated within the body (its 'uptake and distribution');
▓ what the organ does with the radiopharmaceutical – i.e. indicating its function; and
▓ how the radiopharmaceutical leaves the body – its 'clearance'.

Some similarity may be recognised between the gamma rays emerging from the body during an RNI examination, and the emergent beam during a diagnostic X-ray examination. But there are also some fundamental differences.

Image identification

Because the gamma radiation has not passed through the body (from one side to the other) RNI images are in no way similar to radiographic projections. The image shows the distribution of radiation energy emitted from the body's surface (e.g. anterior or posterior) nearest to the gamma camera.

Image unsharpness

There is no obvious RNI parallel to the insistence in diagnostic X-ray imaging, on producing images free from movement unsharpness. During an RNI examination, the patient remains still but not motionless; gamma rays are emitted from the body and measured by a detection device over a period of time measurable in minutes and hours, while the collected energy is translated into an image. There is a clear difference between this arrangement and the millisecond X-ray exposures used in diagnostic radiography.

Similarly, use of a very small X-ray tube focal spot, to reduce geometric unsharpness, cannot be replicated during RNI procedures: the gamma radiation originates within a relatively large area. Instead, the sharpness of a gamma camera image relies on accurate

identification of the emitted photons' origins, by means of a collimator located at its (input/detection) front. The camera's resolution
varies according to the specific type of collimator. High resolution
is not always the primary consideration; echoing the situation
encountered in other imaging modalities, resolution conflicts with
sensitivity. So, when rapid acquisition is essential, such as for
dynamic cardiac studies, a sensitive collimator is selected, and a
degree of resolution is sacrificed.

The gamma camera

Principle

The image receptor within a gamma camera is a large scintillation
crystal, in the form of a flat disc, normally about 1-centimetre thick.
Its outer (front) surface is positioned facing and close to the patient's
body, to absorb the emerging gamma ray photons. The crystal converts absorbed gamma radiation into light energy: each photon produces a flash of light – a scintillation – with brightness directly
proportional to the energy of the detected photon.

The crystal's inner (rear) surface is optically coupled to an array
of 60 or more photomultiplier tubes (see Figure 6.2). These detect
the scintillations and convert their light energy into measurable
electrical signals, proportional to the absorbed gamma ray energy.
The crystal's thickness ideally allows complete absorption of
gamma ray energy but minimal absorption (obstruction) of light.
Signals from the photomultiplier tubes are amplified and fed to a
computer that measures their intensities, and identifies their loca-
tions. The collected data can be analysed and manipulated to construct images based either on overall spatial distribution or (because
detection is continuous) on how the emission of radioactivity
changes with time – 'dynamic studies', that show the sequence of
function in each part of the organ being examined. The choice
between these options depends on which, in a given situation, offers
the more reliable diagnostic information.

Equipment

The crystal and the photomultiplier tubes are sealed into a lightproof aluminium housing that is surrounded, except at its input
surface, by lead shielding. In front of the crystal is a multi-hole,
honeycomb-pattern collimator, usually about 2.5-cm thick (deep),

Six

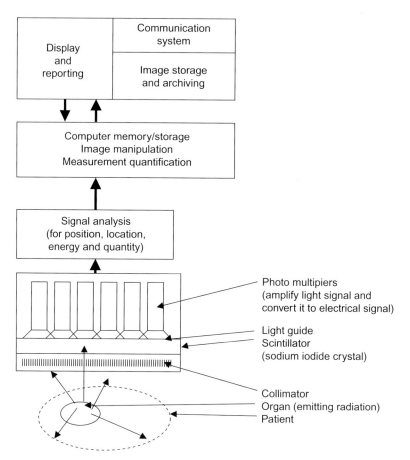

Figure 6.2 Principles of gamma camera operation. Gamma radiation approaching the collimator at 90° passes through to produce scintillations in the sodium iodide crystal. These are detected, amplified, and digitised to form a signal, which passes to the computer.

with septa (dividing walls) constructed of finely-cast lead. Photons travelling along perpendicular paths are allowed to reach the crystal through the collimator's parallel, open channels, but their lead walls restrict access by oblique photons. This selective effect makes the camera direction-sensitive: it allows the origins of the photons to be identified. (It is similar to the action of a secondary radiation grid that allows transmission of aligned primary X-rays but absorbs angled scatter.)

Collimators can be changed, so that septal thickness and the distribution and depth of the holes suit different imaging requirements and photon energies. For radionuclides with higher photon energies, thicker septa (up to 2.5 millimetres) are required, to prevent

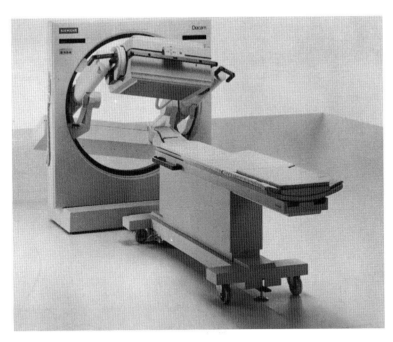

Figure 6.3 Gamma camera and couch. The rectangular gamma camera, mounted in its gantry, is balanced by an equally massive counterweight, located behind. (Photograph by courtesy of Siemens plc.)

radiation from penetrating into adjacent holes. But increased septum thickness reduces sensitivity: it places more lead in the path of the photons, reducing access to the crystal. Similar conflict arises when, in order to increase spatial accuracy, deeper holes are used: access is narrowed, so that photons deviating by more than a small angle from the perpendicular (in relation to the collimator's face) are absorbed by the septa. (This echoes the conflict encountered in X-ray imaging, where gains in image resolution are often only achieved at the expense of speed, and *vice versa*.)

A gamma camera head is extremely heavy, so it is supported on a strong gantry, counterbalanced or motor-driven to allow easy, accurate positioning (see Figure 6.3). Cameras may have a single head but are often dual-headed, with angular adjustments, configuring them to suit anatomical and detection requirements. The patient lies on an adjustable-height, cantilevered support couch with a strong, radiolucent top, allowing the gamma camera head to be positioned as close as possible to the patient. Some gamma cameras are capable of acquiring longitudinal scans and sectional images by appropriate movement of the camera head during acquisition.

Patient care and management

RNI procedures are 'safe': they involve little or no patient discomfort and do not require the use of anaesthesia. But strict regulations governing use of ionising radiation (keeping doses *As Low As Reasonably Practicable*) must be observed.

Lacking the on / off facility with which X-rays are generated, RNI is subject also to legislation and codes of practice governing unsealed sources of radioactivity. These cover the transport and handling of radionuclides, and the prevention of contamination, both of personnel and the environment.

Future developments

RNI is being extended by use of a wider variety of radiopharmaceuticals, different methods of detection, and advanced computer imaging software. Radionuclides that emit positrons are being used to label substances readily absorbed into the body, such as glucose. A type of sectional imaging, *positron emission tomography*, can be performed through use of equipment constructed on principles similar to X-ray computed tomography – and dual-purpose scanning equipment, for both X-ray CT and Emission CT, is being deployed.

Six

Chapter 7
Ultrasound imaging

Introduction

Two similarities link the principles of X-ray and ultrasound imaging:

(1) a beam of energy is directed into the patient's body; and
(2) images are based on how this energy is attenuated by the various body tissues.

But when an ultrasound beam is directed into the patient's body, images are formed by energy *reflected towards the source*, not (like X-rays) transmitted through to a separate image receptor.

Ultrasound imaging can quickly reveal information about the body that would be difficult or impossible to obtain with X-rays, particularly where soft-tissue differentiation is required. Images are formed in 'real time' on a computer screen. This immediate response is essential because an examination's progress depends on feedback to the operator. Certain body planes and beam angulations are known in advance to have diagnostic potential but an ultrasound procedure is essentially operator-dependent. Reliance on skeletal landmarks is relatively minor, so there is no real equivalent to diagnostic radiography's standardised system of projections. If ultrasound imaging is at all comparable to an X-ray procedure, it resembles fluoroscopy, not radiography. But a crucial difference between X-rays and ultrasound weakens this comparison: ultrasound is not an electromagnetic radiation. So, despite absorption of energy into the patient's body there is no possibility of ionisation; elaborate protection for patients and staff is unnecessary. The feasibility of harm is recognised: precautions are enforced; but ultra-sound examinations are normally considered to be relatively 'safe'.

The nature of sound and ultrasound

Sound energy travels through a medium (gas, liquid or solid) as a series of waves, produced by some form of mechanical vibration – a plucked guitar string, for example, or a ringing bell. A medium is essential because sound waves need particles to receive and transmit their energy; they cannot, unlike X-rays, cross a vacuum. The particles vibrate backwards and forwards *along* the path of the wave, subjecting the material to compression, followed by rarefac-tion (stretching) in harmony with the passing wave. This type of response classifies sound as a *longitudinal* waveform (see Figure 7.1).

Sound waves are detected as vibrations by the ear and identified by the brain, according to their intensity (loudness) and pitch. The tympanic membrane's vibration is conveyed to the auditory nerves via a chain of bones, the auditory ossicles. This action reveals the difference between *sound* and *ultrasound*: it is due to the sound's frequency – i.e. the rate at which vibrations occur. The upper limit of human hearing stands at about 20 kilohertz (20 000 cycles per second). Above this, the ossicles are unable to respond: the vibra-tional rate becomes too fast, so sound waves remain unheard. Some forms of hearing deterioration – as an accompaniment to ageing, for example – further limit a person's response, so that 'audible' sounds become inaudible. But ultrasound can broadly be defined as *high-frequency sound, above the detection threshold of the human ear*. Apart from audibility, most features of sound also relate to ultrasound.

Some definitions (see Figure 7.2)

Intensity

The *intensity* of an ultrasound beam expresses the rate of flow of energy. If it were audible, this would be appreciated as loudness. It is directly similar to the intensity of an X-ray beam and the bright-ness of visible light.

Frequency

This is a measure of the rate at which vibrations occur. The unit, indicating the number of cycles per second, is the *hertz* (Hz) or more usually its multiple, the megahertz (MHz = one million hertz).

Seven

(a) Molecules at rest in their natural, regular positions

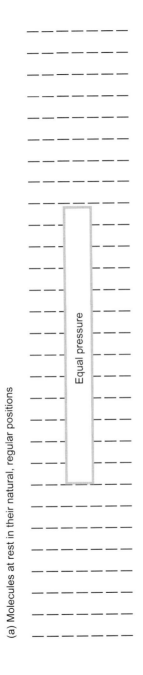

Equal pressure

(b) Molecules displaced longitudinally during the passage of a sound wave

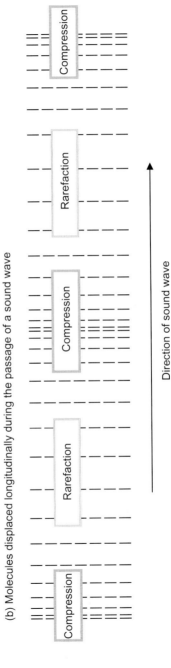

Compression   Rarefaction   Compression   Rarefaction   Compression

Direction of sound wave

Figure 7.1 Schematic representation of sound transmission. Sound energy alternately forces the molecules closer together and pulls them wider apart.

Seven

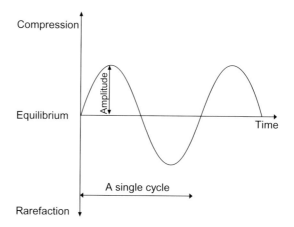

Figure 7.2 Graphical representation of a sound wave. Amplitude is a measurement of the molecules' displacement from their equilibrium positions.

Wavelength

An ultrasound beam's wavelength indicates the separation between successive pulses. It is measured using a unit of length that, depending on the particular sound, may be the metre or the millimetre.

Speed

When travelling through a given medium, the speed of sound is constant, and independent of frequency. If the frequency changes, there is a reciprocal or inverse change in wavelength, so their product remains constant.

Speed, frequency and wavelength are related by the equation:

speed of sound (c) = frequency (f) multiplied by wavelength (λ)
$$c = f \times \lambda.$$

Production and detection of ultrasound

Like X-radiation, ultrasound is produced by conversion of another form of energy. Conversion occurs within an ultrasound *transducer*. This device is a crystal of a *piezoelectric* material [pronounced 'peetso–electric' and literally meaning 'pressure electricity'] that has two essential properties.

(1)   When a voltage is applied across the opposing faces of a piezoelectric crystal, it deforms, as if being compressed or squeezed.

This change of shape is sufficient to make the crystal emit ultrasound – a phenomenon termed *electrostriction*, or the *reverse piezoelectric effect*.

(2)   When a piezoelectric crystal is physically compressed, an electrical voltage is created across its opposing faces. This is the *piezoelectric effect*. A beam of ultrasound incident on (and absorbed into) the face of a piezoelectric transducer is sufficient to generate a detectable and measurable voltage.

So, the ultrasound transducer performs a two-way role, converting electricity into ultrasound and ultrasound into electricity. In other words, the transducer acts as both a transmitter and a receiver.

The ultrasound probe

The transducer is normally housed within an ultrasound probe, a hand-held device, connected by an electrical lead to the equipment's control section. The operator directs the ultrasound beam towards the area being investigated, simultaneously watching the monitor screen, assessing and analysing the examination's progress.

In its transmitting mode, the transducer is supplied with a high-frequency, intermittent voltage which produces rapidly-repeated compressions, causing emission of a sequence of very short ultrasound pulses (measured in microseconds). When pulses encounter a reflective surface within the patient's body, some of their energy is returned towards the transducer which, during the brief intervals between pulse production, acts as a receiver. It absorbs the reflected energy and (re)converts it into a proportionate voltage.

It is important that sufficient time is left between pulses for echoes to be received. The transducer's operation is electronically switched, so that it both transmits and receives accurately, without interference.

Seven

Image formation and display

The time interval between emission of an ultrasound pulse from a transducer and its echo's return depends on (a) the speed of sound through the tissue and (b) the distance travelled – effectively, the depth of the interface. So, if the period between the emission of each pulse and the return of its echo(es) can be very accurately measured, the data can be translated into measurement of the depth of

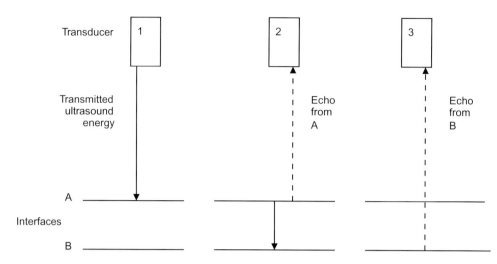

Figure 7.3 Schematic representation of depth localisation. Time periods show: (1) an ultrasound pulse from the transducer (in transmitter mode) travels to interface A; (2) some of the ultrasound energy returns as an echo to the transducer (in receiver mode) while the remainder penetrates to interface B; (3) the delayed echo from interface B returns to the transducer. The time difference between the echoes is translated by the computer into data concerning the interfaces' depths within the body.

the interface(s) from which the energy has been reflected (see Figure 7.3).

When it is operating as a receiver, the transducer collects echo signals; their kinetic energy is proportionally converted into electrical energy, electronically interpreted, and usually displayed as an image on a monitor screen. Owing to the very high rate at which ultrasound pulses are emitted from and received by the transducer, the image information on the screen is updated faster than the human eye can appreciate. This enables movement of the body's internal anatomy to be observed: dynamic, 'real time' images are produced.

Doppler examinations

Doppler ultrasound equipment enables the speed and direction of blood flow to be detected and displayed. The equipment generates ultrasound pulses and contrasts the echoes received from reflectors within the blood moving towards and away from the transducer. Movement produces a characteristic shift in frequency, in the same way that an audible sound moving in relation to a stationary listener (or relatively so) is perceived to change its pitch when approaching movement suddenly changes to receding movement

Seven

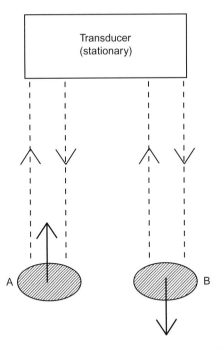

Figure 7.4 Doppler ultrasound. Blood cell A, moving towards the transducer, returns an echo of higher frequency than the original pulse. Blood cell B, moving away from the transducer, reflects a lower frequency signal. Frequency changes are translated by the computer into data concerning the cells' direction and speed.

(see Figure 7.4). (A classic example is heard when an emergency vehicle races past, with its siren sounding.)

Ultrasound interactions

Transmission: acoustic impedance

Unlike X-rays, which are propagated at a constant speed, the speed of sound varies according to the density and compressibility of the material through which it is passing. *Dense* materials, because of their rigidity, allow sound to travel faster than through *compressible* materials, where particles are more energy-absorbent and vibrate more widely, slowing the sound wave's progress.

In clinical practice, despite slight variations in the speed of sound through different organ tissues, a single, average speed of 1540 metres/second is assumed for all body tissues, except bone. Ultrasound equipment is calibrated on the assumption of this average speed.

Seven

Each type of body tissue has an *acoustic impedance*, indicating the opposition it presents to the transmission of ultrasound.

The significance of interfaces

When an ultrasound wave meets an interface (a boundary) between tissues that have different acoustic impedances, some of its energy is returned to the transducer, as an 'echo'. The echo's intensity is proportional to the difference between the tissues' acoustic impedances.

▦   At an interface between two types of soft tissue, because their acoustic impedances *are similar*, only a small amount of energy is reflected to the transducer: i.e. there is a relatively weak signal. Having lost only a small amount of energy, the ultrasound wave is able to progress and generate information about structures, deeper beyond this interface.

▦   Where there is a large *difference* between acoustic impedances, such as at an interface between soft tissue and bone, a relatively large fraction of the energy is reflected to the transducer. The ultrasound wave loses a significant amount of energy, preventing it from returning information about deeper structures. This explains why ultrasound is used extensively to examine soft tissues in the abdomen but has very limited use in relation to soft tissue organs surrounded by bone – for example, the adult brain.

It also explains why a transducer is applied to the patient's skin surface through a layer of gel. By excluding air, the gel enables the ultrasound beam to enter the body with minimal attenuation. Otherwise, owing to differences in their acoustic impedances, an almost total reflection would occur at the interface between air and human tissue. See Figure 7.5.

Angles of incidence

Echo strength depends on another factor: the angle at which the ultrasound beam approaches the interface – the *angle of incidence*.

▦   Reflection at a perpendicular, smooth surface is relatively strong; it is termed *specular* reflection (meaning *as if from a mirror*). A significant amount of the operator's skill is devoted

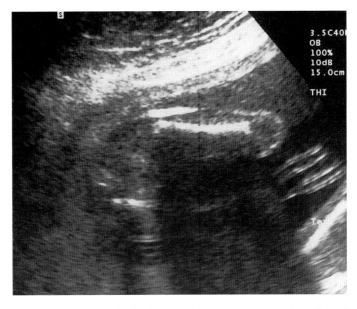

Figure 7.5 Image of a fetal thigh. The transducer is emitting/receiving from the top of the image; the prominent transverse (white) structure is a fetal femur. The large ultrasound reflection at the bone–soft tissue interface casts a shadow distal to the femur, preventing visualisation of soft tissues of the thigh.

to positioning the transducer at exact angles in relation to the shape and orientation of body structures, to achieve specular reflections (see Figure 7.6a).

▪ Where the beam encounters small, irregular surfaces lying at different angles, such as within liver lobules, reflections travel in many directions, forming *scatter* (see Figure 7.6b). In these cases, only a small proportion of the reflected energy returns to the transducer.

These different responses provide information about tissue composition.

Transducer selection

A transducer is selected for an ultrasound examination, to produce the clearest possible image of the required anatomical structure. Two features are central to this choice: image resolution and penetration.

Seven

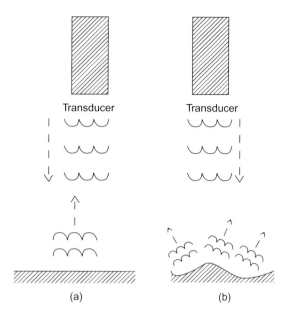

Figure 7.6 Ultrasound interactions at different surfaces. (a) Specular reflection from a smooth interface. The angle of reflection (90°) equals the angle of incidence, and a strong signal is produced. (b) From a rough surface, ultrasound scatters in random directions. The reflection to the transducer is relatively weak, indicating the nature of the tissue (e.g. liver cells).

Image resolution

In common with other imaging modalities, identification of structural detail and pathological change can depend crucially on resolution. More diagnostic information tends to be available if an image has high resolution. Owing to the method by which the ultrasound imaging information is collected, resolution is measurable in two ways.

(1) *Lateral resolution* is the term used for the equipment's ability to distinguish between echoes from small structures lying side by side, across the *width* of the ultrasound beam. The narrower the beam, the greater the lateral resolution. Lateral resolution is optimised by beam focusing: the operator is able to narrow the beam electronically at specific points, along its length.

(2) *Axial resolution* concerns the equipment's ability to distinguish between echoes from two small structures lying close together, one behind the other, *along the length of the ultrasound beam* (i.e. along a dimension at right angles to the lateral resolution plane). Axial resolution increases when pulse length is

shortened – i.e. when higher frequencies are used, shortening the wavelength to 1 mm or less.

Penetration

The amount of penetration required from the ultrasound beam depends on the anatomical structure's location. If it lies deep, like the liver, more penetration is required than for examining a shallow structure such as the eye.

Penetration is a function of the ultrasound beam's frequency. So, a low frequency, between 3 and 5 MHz, is normally used to examine the liver, while for the eye, the frequency is typically 15–20 MHz.

Conflict between penetration and axial resolution

Occasionally, in all imaging modalities, attempts to improve one particular feature of image quality can adversely affect another. These are situations where the skill and experience of the professional staff are particularly needed. In the case of ultrasound imaging, conflict arises when transducer frequency is chosen: higher frequencies improve an image's axial resolution but reduce the beam's penetration – i.e. its ability to provide information about deeper structures.

Conversely, although they provide the best depth penetration, the longer wavelengths associated with low frequencies are less able to resolve smaller echoes – i.e. the image's axial resolution is inferior. In practice, the operator chooses a frequency that strikes a balance between penetration and resolution, offering the optimum diagnostic information.

Positioning the transducer on a part of the body's surface (e.g. anterior, posterior, lateral) as close as possible to the structure being examined, reduces the amount of penetration required. This allows the selected ultrasound frequency to be increased, optimising the image's axial resolution. The success of intracavitary transducers (see below) is based on the relationships between closeness to the structure under examination, ultrasound frequency, and the image's axial resolution.

Types of transducer

Most ultrasound machines offer the operator a choice of at least three different transducers so that, with skill and judgement, the

Seven

most appropriate can be used for each separate examination. Available types vary according to the number of transducer elements they contain, their configuration, size, weight and overall shape, and the sequence in which the separate elements are activated ('fired'). They cater for a whole range of clinical applications. The selected probe should be able to produce images throughout the depth of the area under examination. Multi-frequency probes offer convenience and speed, especially when automatic change is available, linked to the focus depth being used.

▪ A *linear array* transducer is relatively long and narrow, with multiple piezoelectric elements arranged along a straight line (Figure 7.7a). The length of the array determines the width of the field of view. Groups of neighbouring elements are activated sequentially in small groups to transmit and receive echoes, displacing the beam by one element strip each time (approximately 1 mm). So, activation of elements *1 to 10*, is followed by *2 to 11*, then *3 to 12*, and so on. It requires good contact with the skin surface along its whole length (its 'footprint' area) but with parallel beam production and the return signal reception, this type forms images without the need for transducer movement. It is particularly useful for musculoskeletal and vascular applications, where a large field of view is unnecessary.

▪ A *curved array* (*curvilinear*) transducer (Figure 7.7b) has an array of elements that curves outwards. A smaller footprint is required than with the corresponding linear array, but some loss of resolution can occur at the edges of the sector, particularly of structures at lower depths. Element groups are activated in the same way as with a straight linear array, but skin contact is usually easier and the divergent beam increases the field of view. Curved array transducers are extremely popular, particularly for abdominal and for obstetric and gynaecological imaging.

▪ A *phased array* transducer head is very small (typically between 1 cm and 3 cm in width) and constructed from numerous, very thin element strips, packed close together. Their activations are separated by very slight time delays or phase differences, which can be systematically altered electronically, to produce the effect of sweeping the ultrasound field through a sector. Electronic delays are also applied to the subsequent echo signals received at each element. The final echo signal is the sum of the signals from all the elements. These transducers are typically lightweight and easily manoeuvrable. Because the

Seven

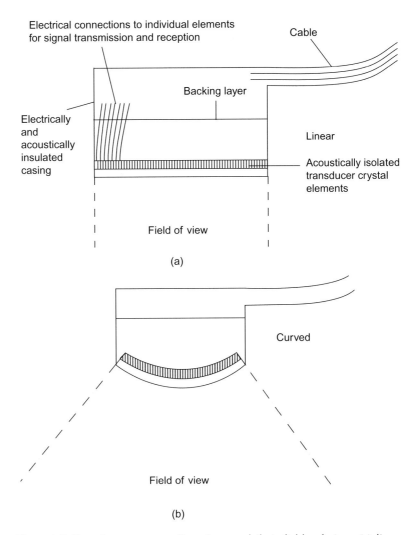

Figure 7.7 Transducer array configurations and their fields of view: (a) linear, (b) curved.

footprint is small, they offer maximum accessibility, particularly where there is only a small acoustic window, e.g. for
cardiac scanning between the ribs, and for neo-natal heads
where access is through the anterior fontanelle.

▦ *Intracavitary transducers* are designed for particular, specialised
applications, such as transvaginal, transrectal and transoe-
sophageal (to examine the heart) procedures. Because these
types of probe can be positioned very close to the area of interest, less penetration is required, so higher frequencies can be
used, to increase image resolution. To illustrate this point: the

transvaginal transducer, which gives optimum image quality in gynaecological examinations and early pregnancy evaluations, operates at frequencies of 5–7 MHz, compared with the 3–5 MHz range used for transabdominal scanning of the same areas. There are disadvantages: it is essential to take precautions to prevent cross-infection; thorough disinfectant cleansing of the probe is required after each examination and disposable covers must be used. These transducers' small footprints limit the field of view but this can be counteracted in some equipment, by the facility of a steerable beam.

▪ *Intraoperative transducers* are very small (perhaps only a few millimetres in diameter) and are usually shaped for specific purposes – for example, for use within catheters for imaging blood vessels. They produce high-quality images through use of high frequencies, up to and exceeding 20 MHz.

Image recording

Several methods of image recording are in use, for both static and dynamic images, from a simple photographic print of the monitor image, to a digital file stored in a computer archive. Each has its advantages – e.g. low cost, or high resolution, or immediate accessibility – and limitations, e.g. need for complex equipment.

Artefacts

As with other modalities, ultrasound images may in some circumstances give false impressions: they can appear to show structures that do not actually exist. Potentially misleading effects include shadowing, duplication and enhancement. Causes include variations in ultrasound velocity that either delay or shorten the time taken for an echo to return; these may be due to ultrasound refraction, reverberation, and interference between pulses. The operator's experience and skill are crucial in distinguishing between authentic image data and artefacts, and in either preventing or compensating for their occurrence.

Safety

Scientific discipline demands a cautious approach to the use of ultrasound: lack of evidence of harm is not assumed to indicate 'safety'. The energy absorbed during ultrasound's transmission through tissues, causing raised vibration of particles, is regarded as a potential source of harm. In contrast to the transmission of X-rays, no ionisation occurs. But as vibrations spread to adjacent particles, so the pressure and density in other areas fluctuate in harmony with the passing wave. Energy is converted into heat, and pressure changes can raise the possibility of biological harm. Risks are known to be associated with ultrasound intensities and frequencies higher than those normally used for diagnostic imaging. These phenomena continue to be investigated, and precautions are taken to ensure that equipment operation remains within defined parameters. For safety reasons, manufacturers are required by law to display thermal and mechanical indices, and power output data on their equipment. But the ultimate responsibility lies with the equipment's operator, to ensure that the amount of energy used for imaging is *as low as reasonably practicable*.

Quality Assurance

Like most of the other energy forms used in imaging, ultrasound cannot be detected by human senses. So a programme of regular checks is necessary, to ensure that the equipment is functioning correctly – for two reasons: to enable image quality to be maintained, and to ensure safety. Standard images of phantoms are produced, and electronic checks are made on the equipment's calibrations.

Future developments

Continuing advances in the processing and manipulation of ultrasound image are increasing the applications of ultrasound in clinical diagnosis. The most critical feature of a medical imaging system is its capacity to provide diagnostic confidence, by maximising image quality. Digital image optimisation is being incorporated, to maintain image quality through all the required depths of tissue – i.e. to address the problem of reduced penetration, which accompanies use of higher frequencies.

Ergonomic features of equipment, such as reduced transducer weight (achieved by using alternative, lighter and more sensitive piezoelectric materials) and increased mobility are receiving attention, in recognition of the operator's working needs – to eliminate repetitive, occupational strains. The benefits of these developments also extend to the patients.

Seven

Improvements in transducers are likely to include replacement of hard ceramic elements with plastic piezoelectric elements, which have greater sensitivity. Arrays operating at higher frequencies will be perfected, and there will be further computerisation of echo signals.

However, ultrasound imaging will remain very much dependent on the skill of the operator, orientating the transducer appropriately, and interrogating the area under examination with a methodical and precise scanning technique.

Chapter 8
Magnetic resonance imaging

Introduction

An MRI examination involves *two* forms of energy. First, the patient is positioned within a very strong magnetic field, to align the body's natural magnetic properties. Then, the anatomical area being investigated is subjected to sequences of very short radio-frequency pulses. Yet, under normal circumstances, provided that strict safety precautions are observed, neither of these can cause harm; so, like ultrasound imaging, MRI is considered to be safe.

During the intervals between the radio-frequency pulses, detectors receive returning signals from body tissues. These are processed by a computer, and converted into detailed, high-resolution images, displayed on the computer's monitor. The signals are produced by *nuclear magnetic resonance*: they are emitted by the nuclei of targeted hydrogen atoms within tissues lying in selected slices through the area being examined. So, magnetic resonance images reveal information about the body, based on the distribution and response of hydrogen nuclei. Their significance, due to the prominence of hydrogen as a constituent of water and fat, gives MRI a particularly important role in demonstrating the body's soft tissues, complementing the skeletal images produced by CT and other X-ray techniques.

The body's magnetic properties

An important step towards understanding MRI is a recognition that the human body has magnetic properties. Popular concepts of magnetism are associated with iron and steel – i.e. with ferromagnetism, and strong forces of attraction and repulsion. Compared with these, the body's magnetic properties seem disappointing: forces are unco-ordinated and weak, and yet they are sufficient for sophisticated MRI scanners to produce detailed, high-resolution images. The derivation of magnetism from an electric current – electromagnetism – is important in many, widely varying situations; its source is the movement of charged particles (electrons) along a conductor. Charged particles are also to be found in motion throughout the body, *within its atoms*. The orbital circulation of negatively-charged electrons around the nucleus generates a magnetic effect too weak to use for MRI. But there is greater potential within the atoms' nuclei, where the positively-charged particles, the protons, spin on their axes. In most atoms, where the numbers of protons and neutrons are equal (i.e. where the mass number is twice the atomic number) and both are even numbers, even this motion is unable to produce a detectable magnetic field, because other nuclear particles exert a cancelling effect. But magnetic effects *can* be detected in atoms where the total number of protons plus neutrons is odd, or where there are odd numbers of both protons and neutrons. Here, the whole nucleus has a spin; so, because of its positive charge (due to the protons) it has a magnetic property, usually termed a *magnetic moment*.

Most elements exist in several isotopic forms: they have a common atomic number but different mass numbers. So the element itself isn't a reliable guide to whether its nuclei have a magnetic moment and MRI significance. For example, the nucleus of an atom of carbon 12, the most common isotope (nuclide) of carbon, contains six proton–neutron pairs (i.e. twelve particles). This nucleus has no magnetic moment. But the nucleus of the *carbon 13* nuclide, with its extra (unpaired) neutron, has a magnetic moment and is MRI-detectable.

Only a limited number of elements display significant magnetic properties but MRI is both feasible and successful because this shortage is offset and outweighed by two key facts about hydrogen.

(1) Its most common isotopic form (accounting for over 99% of the atoms) has a nucleus consisting solely of a proton, so it has a magnetic moment.
(2) It is abundant throughout the body, notably as a constituent of water and fat.

So, MRI is targeted on the hydrogen nucleus because sufficient responsive 'MRI-susceptible' nuclei are found within the body, even

Eight

though in some parts, such as in cortical bone, their MRI suscepti-bility is reduced, due to the hydrogen atoms' chemical bonding.

A spinning nuclear particle shows the magnetic characteristics of a *dipole*: like a bar magnet, its magnetism is concentrated at poles (north/south) at each end of its rotational axis. So, it needs to be explained why the human body as a whole does not normally display magnetic behaviour. The reason is that the axes of the nuclei – and their magnetic fields – are dispersed at random angulations throughout the body. Thus, their effects are mutually cancelling, with no overall effect. This fact may also be expressed by saying that there is no *net magnetic vector* – i.e., the atoms together produce no coherent, unified, directional magnetic force.

The external magnetic field

The first stage of MRI is an alignment of the body's susceptible atomic nuclei, so that their magnetic properties become co-ordinated. This is achieved through the action of the external magnetic field.

Normally, in modern clinical practice, a superconducting magnet is employed to produce the required conditions. Early MRI scan-ners operated with either a permanent magnet or a conventional electromagnet. These had positive features but their operation was also restricted, and both types are now effectively obsolete. A brief look at the restrictions will help to explain why superconducting magnets have become standard.

A huge 'horseshoe' type of permanent magnet produced a stable magnetic field that could be maintained without the need for an energy supply. Inherent field strength tended to be relatively low. It could be raised by increasing the magnet's size and weight, but this led to magnets tending to be extremely heavy, creating installation problems.

An electromagnet, which has its field created by the energy of an electric current, is not as heavy as a permanent magnet and its mag-netism can be switched on and off, as required. Field strength is directly proportional to the electric current that flows through its spiralling, solenoidal windings – so a stronger field can be achieved by increasing the current. But the *current:field strength* relationship does not remain constant. The flowing electrons that form the current through the magnet's windings collide with the conductor's vibrating atoms – the phenomenon of electrical *resistance*. These col-lisions convert electrical energy into heat: the magnet's temperature tends to rise. This aggravates the situation because, having more

Eight

kinetic (vibrational) energy, the conductor's atoms present greater opposition to the current – i.e. the resistance increases. So, an increase in the electrical energy input rate raises the magnet's temperature and reduces its efficiency. This type – termed a 'resistive' electromagnet – presented two problems: it was expensive to maintain, due to the requirement for a high electrical energy input; and it required a water-cooling system, to restrict it to room temperature.

Temperature fluctuations made the magnetic field strength unstable, with consequent effects on the consistency of image quality.

Superconducting magnets

An effective way of removing the limitations caused by an electromagnet's resistance is drastically to reduce its operating temperature – not simply by ordinary cooling methods but by taking the solenoid down to temperature values far below ordinary conceptions of 'cold'. Temperature reduction to 0 K (minus 273°C) would eliminate kinetic energy and electrical resistance, so that a high magnetic field strength could be maintained without a requirement for electrical energy. Near-achievement of these conditions forms the principle underlying the superconducting MRI magnet.

The solenoid coils are located within a heavily insulated chamber, built according to the principle of a vacuum flask. They are cooled to a temperature nearly as low as 0 K through the action of a 'cryogen bath' of liquid helium. Insulation both prevents refrigeration of the room environment – the patient does not feel cold – and restricts the return of liquid helium to its gaseous state, although a very slight amount of 'boiling off' occurs (typically 1% every four or five days), so regular replenishment is needed, by specialist MR engineers.

Superconducting magnets are expensive to purchase but their operating costs are relatively limited; and they enable higher magnetic field strengths to be produced. This, in turn, produces a more homogeneous field: higher-resolution images; reduced scan times; less movement; repeat measurements image quality; improved signal-noise ratio.

Two units are used for measuring magnetic field strength, the gauss (symbol, G) and the tesla (symbol, T). They are related by a factor of 10^4:

$$1 \text{ gauss} = 0.00001 \text{ tesla}$$
$$1 \text{ tesla} = 10000 \text{ gauss } (10\,kG).$$

In normal clinical practice, a superconducting magnet produces a field strength of 0.2–3 T. (The Earth's magnetic field is 0.6 G or 0.000006 T.)

Control of the magnetic field

The magnetic field is carefully controlled, to ensure that:

▪ it is internally homogeneous – i.e. of equal strength throughout – so that imaging processes can be performed accurately, to produce images of the highest quality; and
▪ any external influences, through its 'fringe field', are minimised: shielding is used to protect adjacent structures and personnel.

Shimming

Strength variations, *inhomogeneities*, can be due either to imperfections in the magnet coils' spacing and configuration, or to external influences – e.g. through magnetisation of the steel structure (the yoke) that supports the magnet, or other features within or outside the room. Compensation for these effects, to restore field uniformity, is an important feature of the equipment installation process. It involves a procedure termed *shimming*. *Shim coils*, carrying finely controlled electric currents that create supplementary magnetic fields, are positioned in the vicinity of the main magnet. Their purpose is to restrict main field inhomogeneities, for clinical imaging purposes, to between 5 and 10 *parts per million* (the arbitrary unit in which inhomogeneity is measured).

Fringe field control

The ideal situation, where the magnetic field is totally confined to the patient's body, is impossible to achieve with high field imaging. In practice, it strays outside, forming a *fringe field*. The potential effects of a fringe field are taken into account when MRI magnets are sited: magnetic shielding is employed – either in a *passive* form, through the construction of physical barriers, or an *active* form, by use of additional solenoid magnets to set up opposing (cancelling) fields.

A third type of magnetic field control, the use of *gradient coils*, is described below, in the section concerned with the imaging procedure.

Eight

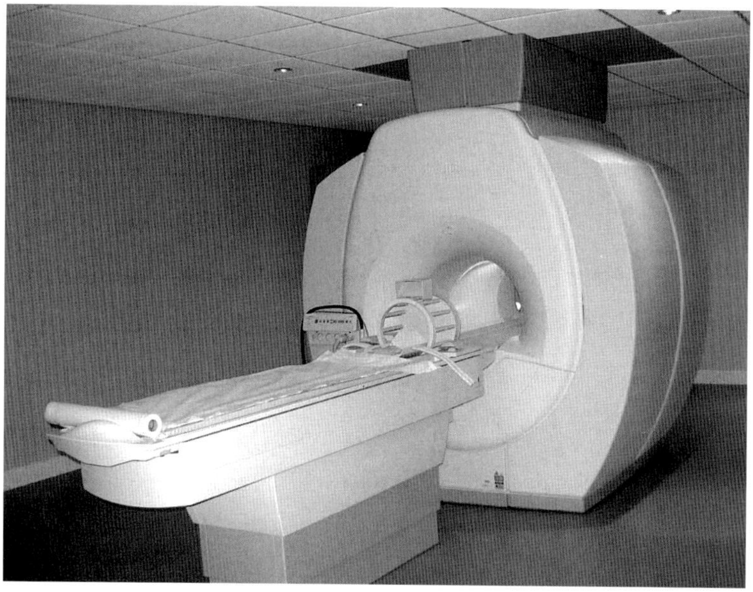

Figure 8.1 A modern MRI scanner. The transmit/receive quadrature head coil is shown in position on the scanner couch. (Photograph by courtesy of Philips Medical Systems.)

Purpose and effect of the external magnetic field

During an MRI examination, the patient lies on a non-magnetic couch, positioned on a track running through the open centre – the *bore* – of the magnet (see Figure 8.1). The patient is moved through the bore, to the isocentre – i.e. the point where all the magnetic gradients intersect, making it the most homogeneous part of the field.

The familiar north–south alignment of a compass needle illustrates the behaviour of a freely-suspended bar magnet within an external magnetic field: it orientates itself and adopts a steady position, with a matching polarity. Despite its comparison to a bar magnet, a spinning nuclear particle does *not* respond in exactly the same way. There are two important differences.

(1) Because of its spinning motion, a nuclear particle does not passively line up along the external field (lines of force). The particle's *mean axis* becomes aligned but its continuing spin makes the particle wobble: one of its poles is in a constant position but the other traces a circular path. This action is termed *precession*. (See Figure 8.2.)

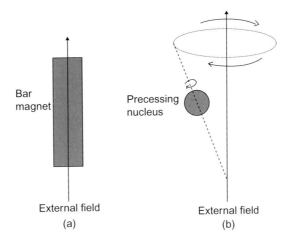

Bar
magnet

External field

(a)

Precessing
nucleus

External field

(b)

Figure 8.2 Precession. Both a bar magnet (a) and a magnetically susceptible nucleus (b) respond to an external magnetic field. A bar magnet moves into stable, stationary alignment but a nucleus precesses: its mean axis is aligned to the field but it continues to show rotational motion.

(2)   Responding, susceptible protons precess with their mean axes in alignment *either along or directly opposed to* the external field (Figure 8.3). This strange behaviour is due to the fact that a proton, though extremely small, is not a fundamental atomic particle: it is composed of smaller particles, e.g. quarks. These determine a proton's energy state in response to the external field: either a low-energy state, in which case it lies parallel to the field, or a high-energy state, where its alignment is termed *anti-parallel*, in opposition to the external field. When alignment occurs, the incidence of these two states tends to be almost equal, but protons in the *lower*-energy state, lying in *parallel* alignment, are in a slight majority.

The imaging procedure

Before imaging begins, the required anatomical area is enclosed in a receiver or surface coil, ready to detect the MRI signals that will be produced by the targeted hydrogen nuclei. These are comparatively weak, so a receiver coil must meet the following criteria.

▨   It must allow positioning as close as possible to the area being imaged, in order to detect the MR signals at their strongest. (Signal strength reduces as distance from the coil increases.)

Eight

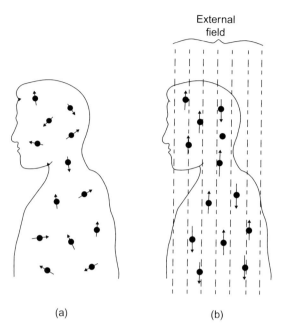

Figure 8.3 The body's response to a strong external magnetic field. From their naturally random arrangement, with no overall magnetic field (a), the body's' nuclei are aligned by a strong external magnetic field (b) – some anti-parallel but a majority in parallel alignment.

- It must have high sensitivity. This clearly brings an advantage but it can also raise a problem through picking up 'noise' (random energy) in addition to the MR signal. Ideally, the signal-to-noise ratio (SNR) should be high.
- It must have a size and shape closely matching the tissue volume being imaged. The area is restricted to the circumference of the coil, whilst the depth (into the patient) from which signals are received is determined by the coil's radius. Close matching restricts noise pick-up to the imaged area only – not from the rest of the body – to enhance the SNR.

To meet these requirements, appropriate specialised receiver coils are normally used – e.g. for imaging the knee, wrist or cervical spine. They are positioned close to the patient's skin but not directly touching it (to guard against the potential effects of heating). These coils achieve a high SNR and produce high-resolution images but positioning in relation to the patient is critical, some (notably, a head coil) can make patients feel claustrophobic, and their anatomical coverage is restricted. Coverage of larger areas, such as the chest and abdomen, can be achieved by the use of *phased array* coils – multiple, small coils, grouped together, with their signals integrated to give a single high-resolution image and a high SNR.

Signal generation

When the patient is positioned on the couch within the homogeneous magnetic field, the susceptible hydrogen atoms' nuclei within the body precess.

Just over half of the precessing hydrogen nuclei are in a low-energy state, in a parallel orientation; the remainder, in a high-energy state, are in anti-parallel alignment. The effect of alignment is to combine the magnetic effects of the nuclei into two opposing forces – (1) along and (2) in opposition to the external field. Although the difference is slight, the majority of parallel nuclei cancel out the opposing minority, to produce a small, overall longitudinal force, termed the *net magnetisation vector* (NMV).

Two facts about this longitudinal NMV are particularly significant:

(1)   because it is in equilibrium with the external field, and millions of times weaker, it is *undetectable*; and

(2)   It represents only *part of* the magnetic energy of the precessing nuclei. In a similar position, the NMV of aligned, parallel bar magnets would represent 100% of their forces. These two situations and their effects are different due to the precession of the nuclei.

As well as a longitudinal component, each precessing nucleus produces a transverse component. The transverse components of the nuclei as a whole have no detectable effect, for a reason similar to the lack of an overall magnetic effect from the nuclei dispersed throughout the body before the external field is imposed. Individually, they act randomly; so, their effects cancel each other out. In this case, the random factor concerns the direction of the rotational angles of the nuclei: their precessions are normally unsynchronised, or *out of phase*. The reason is that each nucleus is in a local equilibrium: it is responding to and demonstrating the influences of its immediate surroundings.

To summarise: positioning of the patient within the strong magnetic field does not, by itself, yield information that can be converted into an image. The precessing nuclei:

■   exert a longitudinal net magnetisation vector but this is undetectable because it is in equilibrium with the much stronger applied external field;

■   cannot exert a combined transverse magnetic component because their precessional motions are out-of-phase with each other.

Eight

Radio-frequency transmission

RF transmitter coils tend to be large, to produce uniform field coverage and excitation. The main coils are the body coil (used for most imaging examinations) and the head coil. Simultaneously with RF pulse transmission, three gradient magnets (see below) are activated, to modify the magnetic field locally, to cover the thin sections selected for imaging.

Two important terms

Precessional (Larmor) frequency

The number of times a nucleus precesses (i.e. completes one circular wobble) in one second is termed its precessional frequency (or Larmor frequency, after the scientist who pioneered investigation into nuclear magnetic resonance). This is an important, distinguishing characteristic of a particular element (isotope) but it *also depends on the strength of the applied magnetic field* increasing as the field becomes stronger. In a magnetic field of uniform strength, all the nuclei of a given element precess at the same frequency.

Resonance

This is an energy exchange process that uniquely occurs when there is a coincidence between the parameters or features of the object and of the incident energy supply (dimensions, wavelength or frequency). In the case of precessing atomic nuclei, electromagnetic radiation energy can be absorbed when its frequency matches their own precessional frequency. For the hydrogen nuclei and the magnetic field strengths used in MRI, this frequency lies within the radio wave region of the electromagnetic spectrum.

The radio-frequency pulse and the body's response

When the frequency of the RF pulse matches their own precessional frequency, precessing nuclei resonate: they absorb its energy. This produces two effects.

(1)   Some nuclei are changed from their low-energy, parallel alignment into a high-energy, anti-parallel orientation (informally, they are said to be 'flipped' through 180°, to point in the opposite direction), changing the longitudinal net magnetisation vector.

Eight

(2) The precessional angular movements of the susceptible nuclei become *phase-coherent*. This unites their transverse magnetic moments, establishing a detectable transverse component of the net magnetisation vector.

These effects are only temporary: they start to fade when the energy supply is withdrawn, i.e. at the end of the RF pulse. Two distinct reversion processes occur simultaneously but independently. The resonating nuclei:

(1) revert to their former, low-energy state, and to parallel alignment; and then
(2) they lose their phase coherence.

These processes are known as *relaxations*. They happen very quickly, occupying only very brief periods, but they are crucial to magnetic resonance imaging. During relaxation, most* of the excess energy is released by the relaxing nuclei in the form of two, separate, detectable radio-frequency signals. In other words: the relaxing nuclei temporarily become RF transmitters. (*The remainder of the released energy can cause localised heating – a hazard that is monitored.)

Detection of the MRI signals

The RF signals detected by the surface coils indicate the rates at which the two forms of relaxation occur. Both processes occur exponentially, so the signals are not timed through to their conclusions. Instead, their changing strength is detected over a sufficient period of time to allow the relaxation rates (i.e. the exponential *time constants*) to be measured accurately. Both indicate how quickly the nuclei are transferring their excess energy into the local environment, and are diagnostically significant.

Longitudinal (spin–lattice) relaxation

The rate at which the relaxing nuclei revert to their parallel alignment, restoring the longitudinal component of the NMV, depends on how quickly the nuclei can transfer their excess energy to the surroundings (the 'lattice'). The time constant, T1, is defined as the time taken for the longitudinal magnetic component to be restored to 63% of its original value (before resonance). This gives

Eight

information about the physical state of the examined tissues: their composition and structure.

Transverse (spin–spin) relaxation

The relaxing nuclei lose their precessional coherence (they 'dephase') at a rate governed by their interaction with each other. While this occurs, the transverse magnetic component, established during resonance, decays. The time constant, T2, is defined as the time taken for the transverse magnetic component to be reduced to 37% of its original value (during resonance). It gives information about the nature of the biochemical environment surrounding the nuclei.

The high contrast of magnetic resonance images is because relaxation times are different for each type of tissue, and whether the tissue is normal or diseased.

Selection of the image slices

A magnetic resonance image presents diagnostic information about a narrow slice through the body. This means that T1 and T2 data must be collected from relaxing nuclei within a limited plane only.

Originally, care is taken to ensure that the main magnetic field is homogeneous throughout the body. But slice selection (i.e. data collection during resonance) employs the fact that, although the precessional frequency of a nucleus is characteristic of its (chemical) element, it is also proportional to the strength of the magnetic field in which it is situated. So, to establish the conditions for slice selection, local field strength must be modified. *Gradient coils* act three-dimensionally to set up field strength gradients in any plane through the body, along the axis of a required sequence of slices. The coils are carefully stabilised and shielded. They operate by imposing a combination of reinforcing and opposing supplementary forces on to the background field, along sagittal, coronal and axial planes. So, within a region where a sequence of slices is required, each plane will acquire a slightly different field strength and *the nuclei within this plane will have a slightly different precessional frequency*, compared with adjacent, parallel planes. The actual difference between adjacent planes will depend on the steepness of the imposed gradient.

The imaging of a selected slice is then achieved by adjustment of the RF pulse to a frequency that exactly matches the precessional

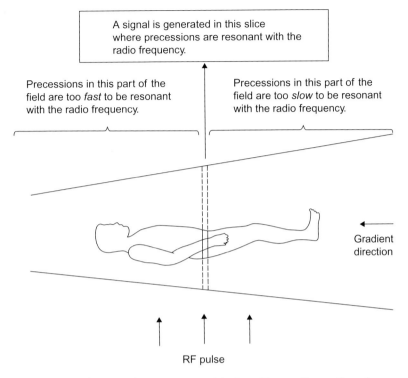

Figure 8.4 Localisation of a transverse axial plane. The gradient coil produces a range of precessional frequencies along the body's axis (here: shorter frequencies to the left; longer frequencies to the right).

The radio-frequency pulse creates resonance within the narrow slice where its frequency matches the local precessional frequency.

frequency of the nuclei within that plane (see Figure 8.4). Resonance will be limited to those nuclei, and their emitted signals will lead to construction of an image of that slice alone. In practice, to display a slice thickness greater than the infinitely thin section that a single, precise frequency would achieve, an RF pulse will comprise a narrow 'band width' of frequencies. So, slice thickness is also dependent on band width, as well as on the gradient's steepness.

The action of gradient coils is under computer control and there is no requirement for the patient's position to be adjusted in any way. The coils are energised to emit pulses to vary field strength at the same time as the RF pulses that produce resonance. The signals are encoded for slice location and identification. (The simultaneous action of the gradient field and the RF pulse is marked by a loud banging noise. The patient must be warned about this beforehand, and provided with ear protection.)

Eight

Imaging control programmes

Computer programmes control the sequence of setting up magnetic field gradients, applying RF pulses and acquiring data for image reconstruction. Separate programmes have been developed to demonstrate particular features and image characteristics. This is a complicated area of MRI practice, which is continuously being developed, as technology advances. The following notes offer an outline only.

The length of the radio-frequency pulse(s)

The RF pulse frequency is matched to the precessional frequency of the hydrogen nuclei, causing them to resonate: some nuclei are raised to the higher energy state, so that they lie anti-parallel, instead of parallel; and the nuclei are made to precess in phase. If the RF pulse's energy is sufficient to (1) remove the longitudinal component by making parallel and anti-parallel forces equal; and (2) create a transverse component (due to the in-phase precession) its overall effect is to change the direction of the net magnetisation vector through an angle of 90°. This may be referred to as a '90° pulse'.

If the RF pulse is longer, so that it reverses alignment of the precessing nuclei into an anti-parallel orientation to an extent that this becomes the direction of the NMV, the pulse may be termed a '180° pulse'. Depending on the relative strength of the longitudinal and transverse components, the NMV may also be moved through other, intermediate angles, depending on the investigation.

Repetition time (TR)

This is the period, measured in milliseconds, between one RF pulse and the next.

Echo time (TE)

This is the period (again, measured in milliseconds) between the RF pulse and the collection of the signal.

Weighting

Spin–lattice and spin–spin relaxation processes occur simultaneously, so images are influenced by both; a pure T1 or T2 image

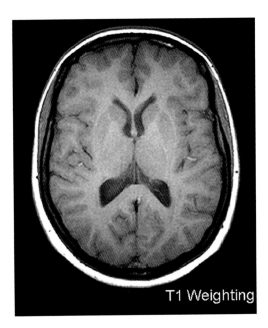

T1 Weighting

Figure 8.5 T1 weighted axial image of the brain. Fat, e.g. subcutaneous fat, appears white (high signal); water, e.g. in the ventricles, appears dark (low signal). (Image by courtesy of the University of Sheffield MRI Unit at the Royal Hallamshire Hospital, Sheffield.)

cannot be obtained. But by employing combinations of 180° and 90° RF pulses and by varying the TR and TE, pulse sequences can construct biased or *weighted* images (see Figures 8.5 and 8.6).

Gating

Magnetic resonance imaging can also employ the technique of *gating* (as used in RNI and other imaging modalities) to record artefact-free images of structures affected by cyclic movement. For example: where the cardiac cycle is involved, a cardiac monitor triggers the MRI sequence at the same point in every cardiac cycle to obtain identical still images.

Safety precautions

The need for precautions must not be interpreted as contradicting the status of MRI as a safe imaging modality: they are concerned with *maintaining* the safety of all persons involved in MRI procedures, patients and staff, and conditions both within the magnet/scan room and its surrounding environment.

Eight

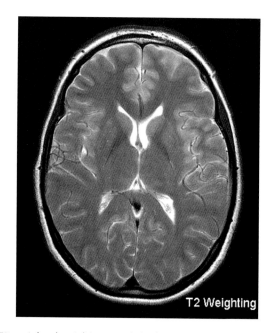

T2 Weighting

Figure 8.6 T2 weighted axial image of the brain. Fat appears dark (low signal); water appears white (high signal). (Image by courtesy of the University of Sheffield MRI Unit at the Royal Hallamshire Hospital, Sheffield.)

Personal safety

The patient

Operational precautions

Used at excessively high energies or levels of intensity, any 'safe' procedure can cross the boundary into becoming potentially dangerous. So, operational limits are imposed by the national and international authorities (who are also responsible for protection from ionising radiations) to restrict technical parameters:

- ▨ the magnetic flux density (field strength);
- ▨ the rate at which magnetic field gradients can be changed; and
- ▨ heating caused by the body's absorption of RF energy.

Contra-indications

MRI requests are subject to some clinical contra-indications.

- ▨ Patients who have certain kinds of metallic implants or surgical clips may be at risk of injury if these devices are moved or deflected by the force of the magnetic field.

- MRI is totally contraindicated for patients with cardiac pacemakers *in situ*. The strong magnetic field will cause a pacemaker to malfunction.
- Metal prostheses may be secure enough to remain safe (if they have been in place for more than 6 to 8 weeks) but they should be observed and the examination halted if the patient feels discomfort.
- MRI is contraindicated for routine examinations during the first 16 weeks of pregnancy unless, in exceptional cases, the clinician believes that the benefit will outweigh the risk.
- Some studies have shown that exposure to strong magnetic fields could cause short-term memory loss.

Before an MRI examination begins

- Every patient must complete an MRI safety screening form to confirm that s/he
  - has had no head or heart surgery,
  - does not have a cardiac pacemaker,
  - has not had a ferromagnetic metallic foreign body in the eye.
- Positive answers to any of these questions may totally contraindicate MRI.
- Patients must remove all metallic jewellery and clothing that contains metallic accessories.
- Credit cards and other similar items which will be 'wiped' by the magnetic field must be deposited in safe keeping, fully shielded from the magnetic field.
- To allay anxiety, the patient must be advised about the loud banging noise that can be expected (when the gradient coils and RF transmitters are simultaneously energised). To add to the patient's well being, ear plugs are supplied.

During an MRI examination

- Communication between staff and the patient is assisted by an observation window from the control room into the magnet/scan room and closed-circuit TV with audio may be provided.
- Having an MRI scan may be a claustrophobic experience for the patient, so an emergency call button is available, to provide an extra feeling of reassurance, and the playing of background music may be helpful.
- Resuscitation equipment must be available but, as this is normally not MRI-safe, resuscitation procedures must take place

Eight

outside the magnet room. Every MRI unit has local rules in place, to ensure this practice is observed.

Other personnel

Because there is no hazard from ionising radiation, friends or relatives may attend the patient, if required, provided they have been screened, like the patient, concerning jewellery, cardiac pacemakers, etc., and are carrying no loose metallic objects.

Outside the times when MRI examinations are being performed, local rules and other protocols, including fire safety procedures, ensure the safety of staff who may be required to enter the magnet room to carry out routine domestic or maintenance work or during emergency situations.

The magnet is never switched off, unless an emergency occurs.

Within the magnet room

The magnetic field

Loose ferromagnetic metallic objects are prohibited. Though of reduced intensity, a shielded fringe field is strong enough to create a serious hazard.

Small objects such as scissors and needles can be snatched off trolleys or out of pockets and drawn through the air at a dangerously high velocity (the 'MRI missile effect').

Larger objects such as wheelchairs, trolleys or resuscitation equipment can present even greater risks, unless they are MRI-compatible (i.e. non-ferrous).

Metal detectors may be installed at entrances to the room, to reinforce prohibition but they have been shown to lack the sensitivity required for detecting all metallic implants.

Cryogenic gas leaks

Where a superconducting magnet is in use, stringent monitoring precautions are required to reinforce the care taken to prevent gaseous leakage of the cryogenic liquid helium. There are two identifiably separate hazards: refrigeration of the magnet's bore and the room atmosphere, and risk of suffocation due to exclusion of oxygen. The low density of gaseous helium will cause it to fill a room from the ceiling downwards, so an oxygen monitor is mounted high in the room, to trigger alarms in case of a helium leak.

If a very serious emergency occurs (e.g. if there is a temperature rise within the cryostat, or if a person is trapped or injured against the magnet), it may prove necessary to terminate the magnetic field. This requires deliberate release of the cryogen, to 'quench' the magnet – and the room's venting system is designed to cope with this rare event.

RF shielding

As well as taking care to prevent the magnetic fringe field from extending outside the magnet room, it is equally necessary to prevent external RF signals from any source, e.g. television and radio transmissions, from *entering*. Even under favourable conditions, the resonant signals emitted by the patient are weak. Without effective screening, interference would contaminate these signals, raise the level of noise, and degrade image quality. The walls, ceiling and floor of the room form a *Faraday* cage – i.e. an RF-shielded cage, made of copper or aluminium. The screening is electrically continuous across all doors, vents, openings for electrical supplies and other services such as piped anaesthetic gases or oxygen passing through a waveguide, and the observation window from the control room.

The external environment

Restricted and controlled areas are clearly defined in the local rules. The magnet's fringe field will have been incorporated in the room design, employing protective distances and shielding, to prevent it from affecting persons or sensitive equipment, such as electron microscopes or image intensifiers, outside the room, including areas above and below. Areas for public circulation are considered safe if field strength is below 5 gauss. But even when precautions have enclosed the 5-gauss line, clear warning signals have to be displayed at entrances to the room to prevent unauthorised entry. There are similarities to the precautions taken to prevent accidental entry of personnel into an X-ray room, but a distinction may be recognised between the *permanent* presence of the magnetic field and the normally intermittent X-ray controlled area.

Quality Assurance

As in other areas of imaging, QA is dually concerned with safety and image quality. Despite being free from the dangers of

Eight

ionisation, MRI quality assurance is still concerned with the bio-logical safety of patients and staff. But the emphasis may be more heavily placed on monitoring the accuracy of equipment concerned with relaxation time measurements, image construction, and the signal-to-noise ratio. Special phantoms should be used daily, to achieve this.

Future developments

The design technology of MR scanners advances continually. Increased 'openness' of whole-body scanners is being pursued, par-ticularly to benefit patients who are prone to claustrophobia. Scan-ners with specialised application – i.e. limited to specific parts of the body – may become cost-effective. Image quality is being improved by advanced design of transmitter and receiver coils; and real-time and whole-body imaging are becoming more accessible.

Further studies

The nature of learning is continuous. Very few resources are in themselves complete: ultimately, they serve as introductions to others – either more advanced, more detailed or more up-to-date. The following are suggested for your further study.

X-ray imaging and general

Books

Ball, J. and Moore, A. D. (1997) *Essential physics for radiographers*, Blackwell Science.

Farr, R. F. and Allisy-Roberts, P. J. (1997) *Physics for medical imaging*, Saunders.

Graham, D. T. (2003) *Principles of radiological physics*, Churchill Livingstone.

Websites

http://www.radiation.org.uk/ (a very useful portal)

http://hpa.org.uk/radiation/ (a government site concerned with safety)

Every manufacturer of imaging equipment has a website – most easily accessed via one of the international search engines using *either* the manufacturer's name and 'medical' *or* a description of the equipment's specialised purpose.

Computed tomography

Books

Kane, S. A. (2001) *Physics in modern medicine*, Taylor and Francis, London.

Seeram, E. (2001) *Computed tomography: physical principles, clinical applications and quality control*, W. B. Saunders, Baltimore.

Silverman, P. M. (2000) *Multislice computed tomography – a practical approach to clinical protocols*, Lippincott, Williams and Wilkins, London.

Website

http://www.comp.leeds.ac.uk/medvis/Info/related_CT.html

Radionuclide imaging

Books

Chandra, R. (1997) *Nuclear medicine physics – the basics (5th edn)*, Lippincott, Williams and Wilkins, London.

Websites

http://www.bnms.org.uk (The British Nuclear Medicine Society)
http://www.ipem.org.uk/ (The Institute of Physics and Engineering in Medicine)

Ultrasound

Books

Fish, P. (1990) *Physics and Instrumentation of diagnostic medical ultrasound*, Wiley.

Zagzebski, J. A. (1996) *Essentials of ultrasound physics*, Mosby.

Websites

http://www.bmus.org (The British Medical Ultrasound Society)

Magnetic resonance imaging

Books

Hashemi, R. H. and Bradley, W. G. (1997) *MRI – the basics*, Williams and Wilkins, Baltimore.

Hennel, J. W. *et al.* (1997) *A primer of magnetic resonance imaging*, Imperial College Press, London.

McRobbie, D. W. *et al.* (2003) *MRI – from picture to proton*, Cambridge University Press.

Westbrook, C. (1998) *MRI in practice*, Blackwell Science.

Shellock, F. G. (2003) *Reference manual for magnetic resonance safety*, John Wiley.

Websites

http://www.mrisafety.com

http://www.mhra.gov.uk (The Medical Devices Agency – with a useful and detailed safety section)

http://www.bamrr.org.uk (British Association of MR Radiographers)

http://www.ismrm.org/smrt (The Section of Magnetic Resonance Technologists in the USA)

Index